THE ULTIMATE REP MAX X2 TRANSFORMATION WORKOUTS

The ULTIMATE REP MAX X2 TRANSFORMATION

WORKOUTS

The Best Isometric Exercises to build muscle, increase strength, burn fat and sculpt the best body with the power of Isometrics!

BECOME A RIPPED!

The Ultimate Rep Max X2 Transformation Workouts was written to help you get closer to your physical potential when it comes to real muscle sculpting strengthening exercises. The exercises and routines in this book are quite demanding, so consult your physician and have a physical exam taken prior to the start of this exercise program. Proceed with the suggested exercises and information at your own risk. The Publishers and author shall not be liable or responsible for any loss, injury, or damage allegedly arising from the information or suggestions in this book.

The Ultimate Rep Max X2 Transformation Workouts
a muscle-building master-plan

By

Birch Tree Publishing
Published by Birch Tree Publishing

The Ultimate Rep Max X2 Transformation Workouts
published in 2020, All rights reserved,
No part of this book may be reproduced, scanned,
or distributed in any printed or electronic form without permission.

Birch Tree Publishing

Dedication

Build Powerful Isometric Muscles **TODAY!**

Contents

A Powerful Body Starts Here

BUILD YOUR BODY "GET" TRANSFORMED

with The Ultimate Rep Max X2 Transformation Workouts the fastest strength-producing program right in the palms of your hands!

Introduction by Marlon Birch CSCS

Trainees of my Bullworker Series" know that I present the best muscle-building programs to increase optimum strength and add quality to one's life. That's my ultimate goal with my muscle enhancing programs.

This book introduces The Ultimate Rep Max X2 Transformation Workouts these programs will get you in the best shape **FASTER** than you thought possible. With the power of our system and the muscle-building benefits of isometrics holds. Combining Isotonics and Isometrics forces the muscles to contract harder and over come neuromuscular system failure.

Our methods extend a set beyond failure, and you will see muscle popping up almost overnight. While getting more muscular and leaner than ever before. It's an eye-opening program that can help you pack on muscle and strength fast. We also look at the optimal rep speed for you to keep building muscles while applying various factors to increase growth.

Keep moving forward

Marlon Birch

Yours In Health and Strength

FULL-BODY WORKOUTS

CHAPTER 1
POWER 5 PROGRAM
PHASE ONE
4 WEEKS
REP SPEED CONTRACT 2 SECONDS, RELEASE 5 SECONDS

01 POWER 5 PROGRAM PHASE ONE

Perform 5 reps, on the 5th rep perform a 20 second Isometric contraction. All exercises are done non stop until one round is finished. Rest 5 seconds between rounds. Alternate day one and day two for 6 days per week.

DAY ONE

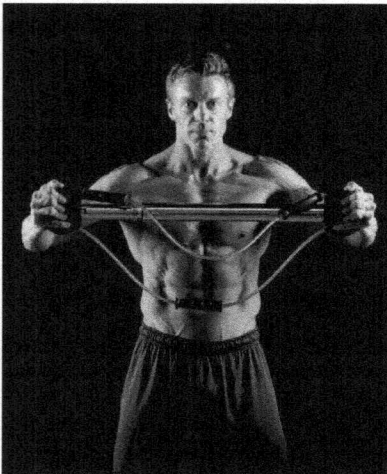
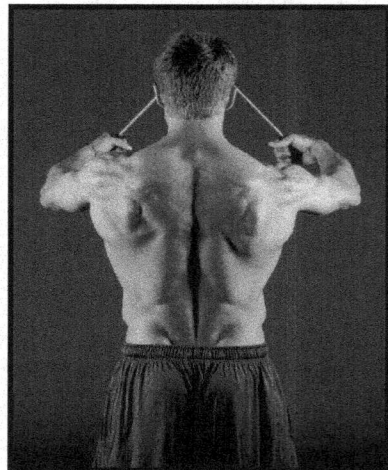
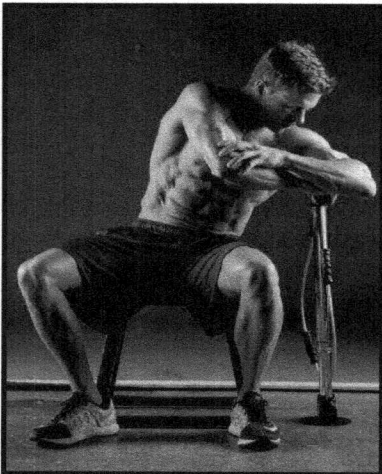
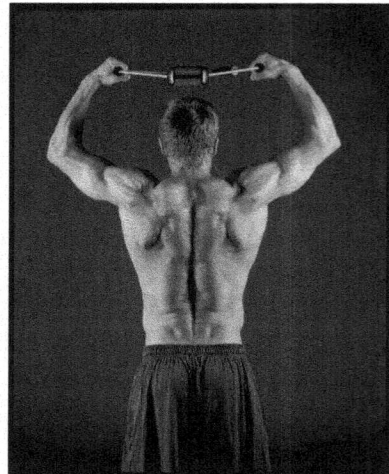

01 POWER 5 PROGRAM PHASE ONE

DAY ONE CONTINUED.....

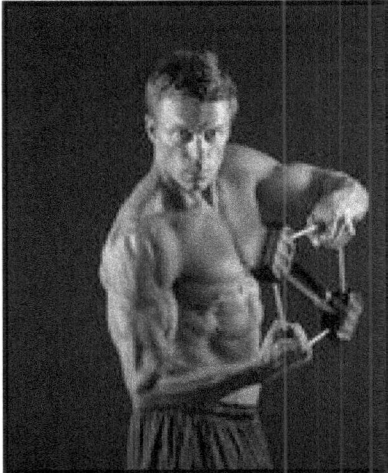

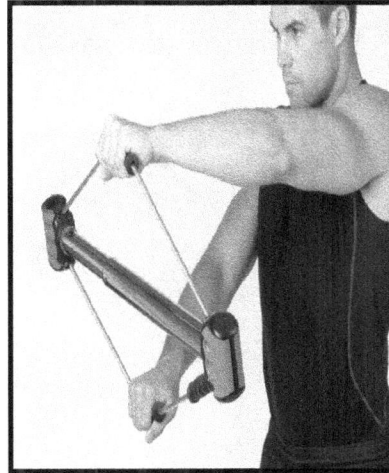

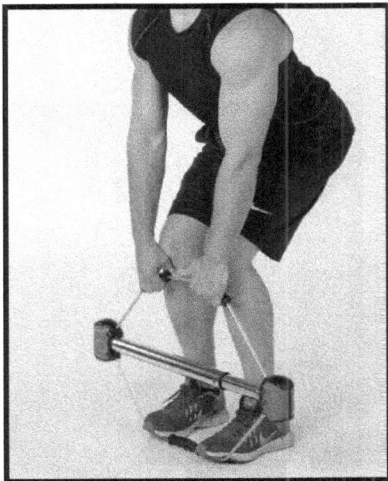

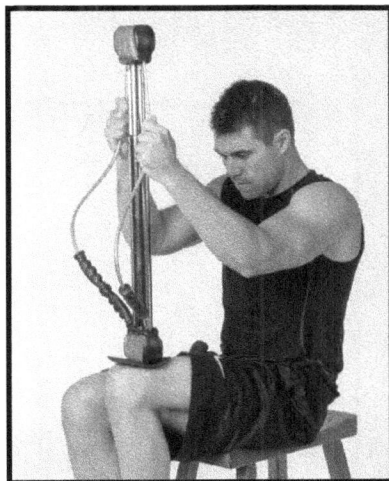

01 POWER 5 PROGRAM

DAY TWO
Same instructions as Day one.

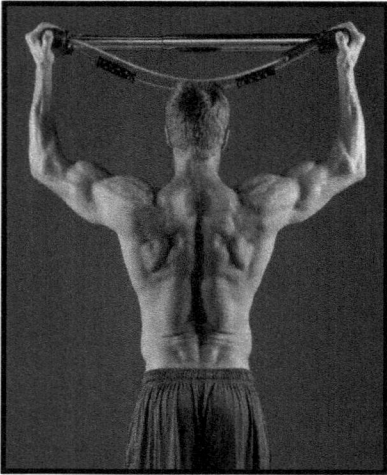

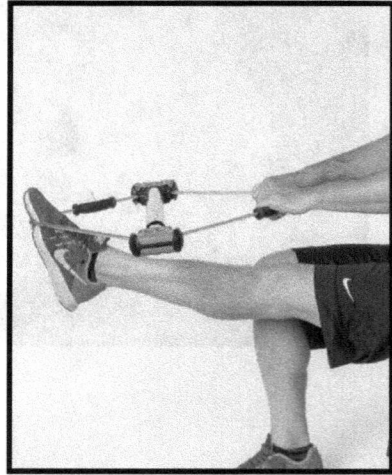

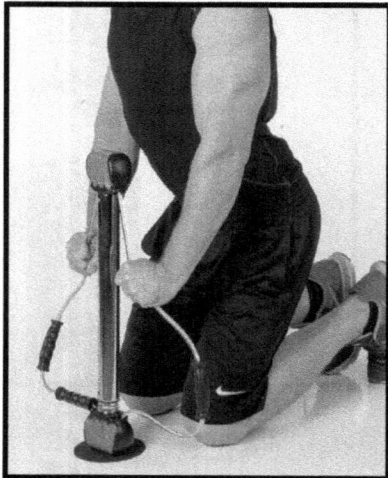

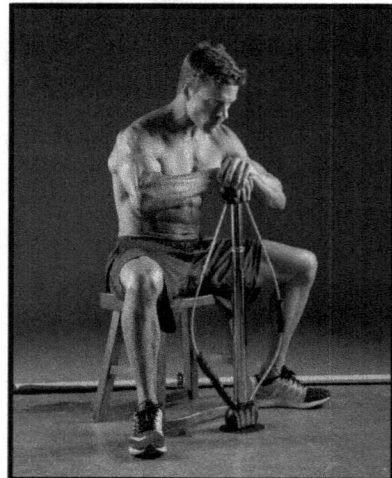

01 POWER 5 PROGRAM
DAY TWO CONTINUED.......

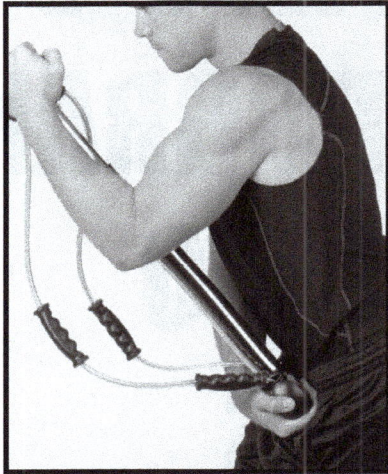

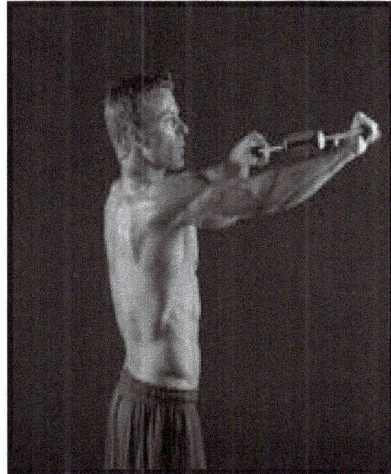

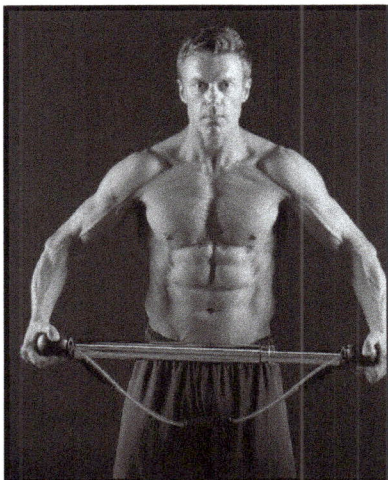

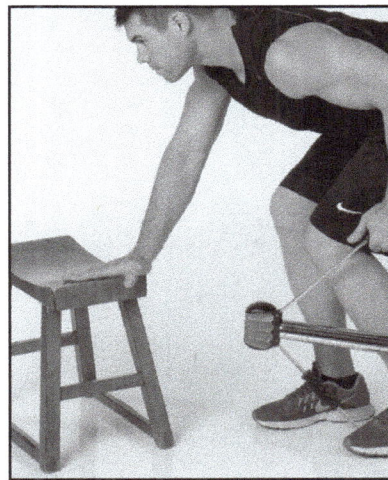

CHAPTER 1
POWER 8 PROGRAM
PHASE TWO
4 WEEKS
REP SPEED CONTRACT 2 SECONDS, RELEASE 2 SECONDS

01 POWER 8 PROGRAM

Perform 8 full reps, followed by 8 half reps. At the start position to the mid-point of the exercise stroke. On the 8th half rep perform a 5 second Isometric contraction. Two sets each exercise. All exercises are done non stop until one round is finished. Rest 5 seconds between rounds. Alternate day one and day two for 6 days per week.

DAY ONE

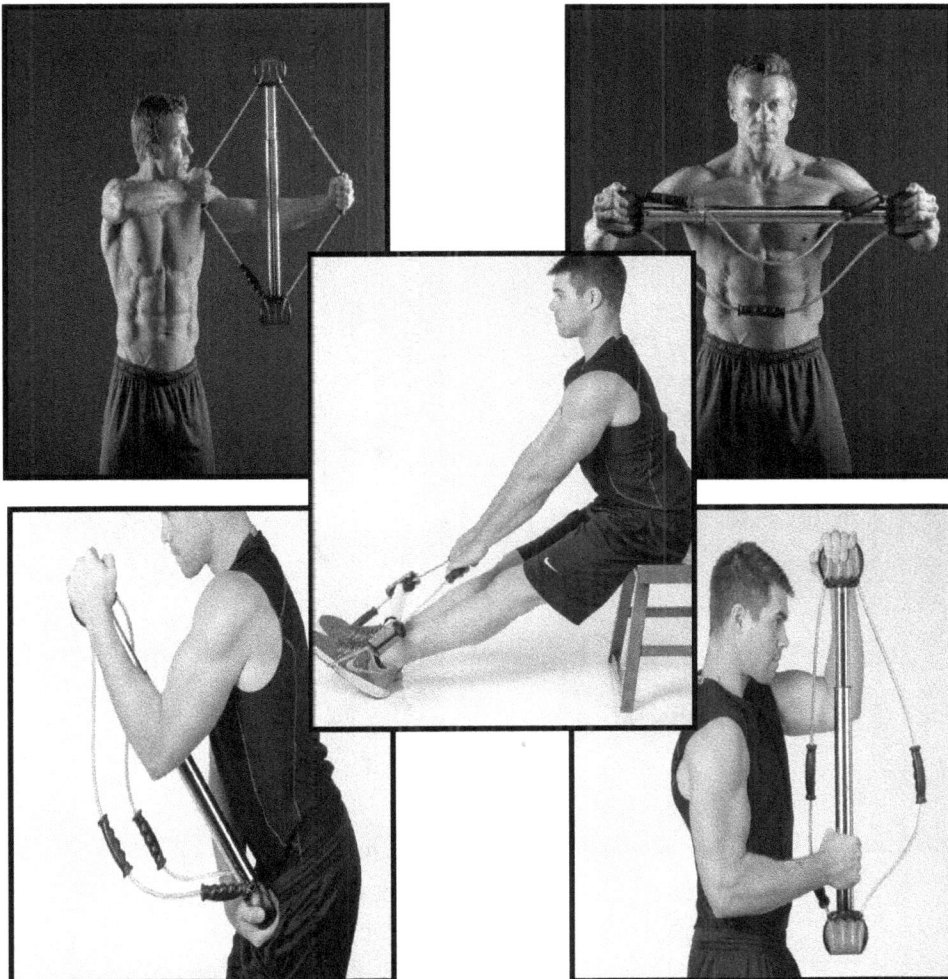

01 POWER 8 PROGRAM

DAY TWO

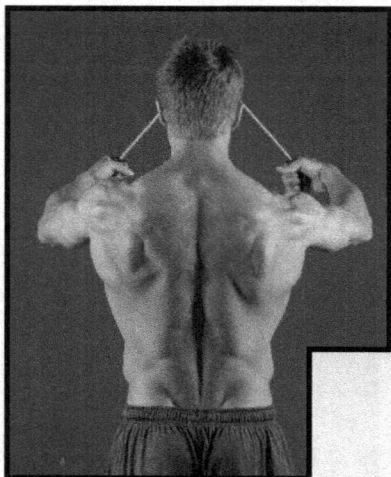
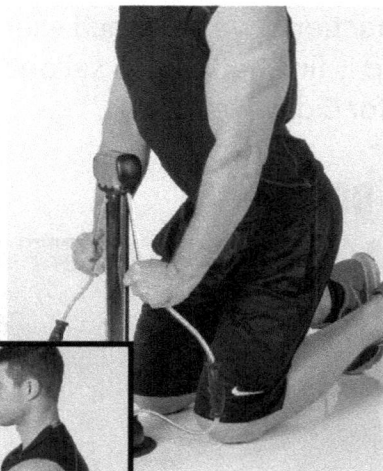
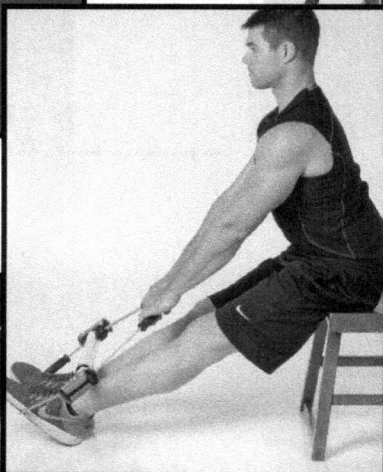
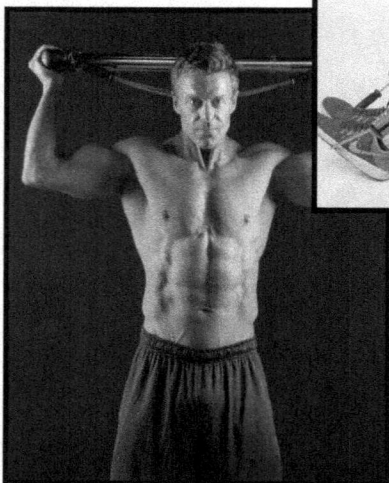
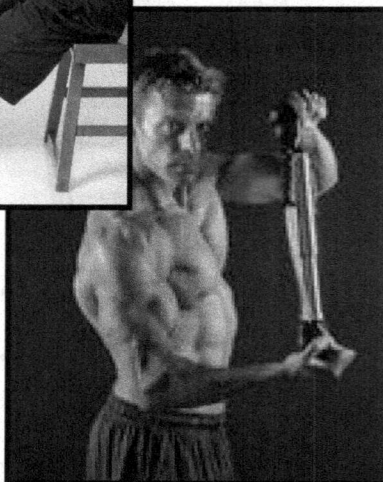

CHAPTER 2

MAX SURGE

PHASE THREE

4 WEEKS

REP SPEED CONTRACT 2 SECONDS, RELEASE 2 SECONDS

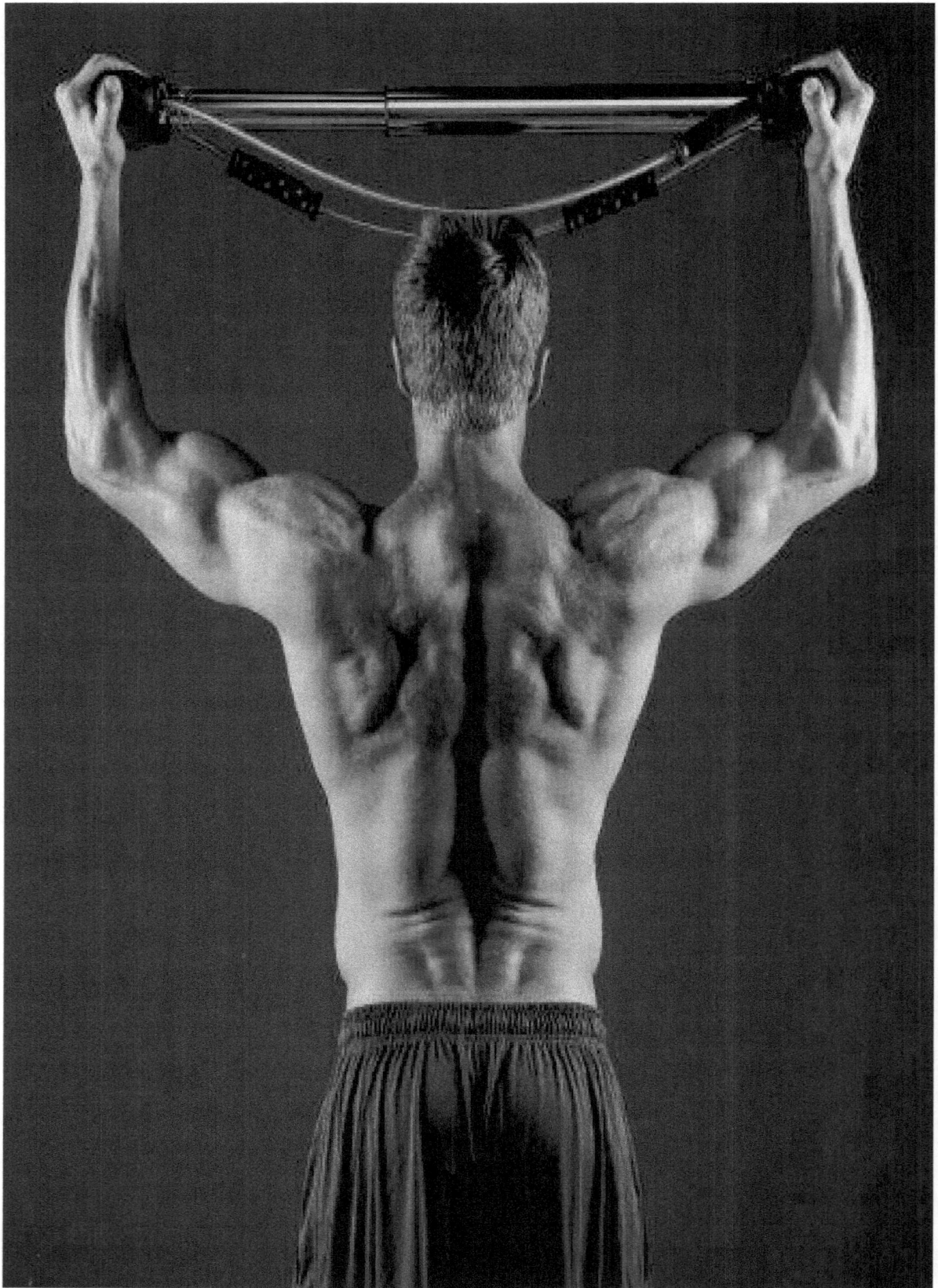

02 MAX SURGE PROGRAM

Perform all exercises non-stop. Perform 7-9 reps per bodypart, on the 9th rep perform a 10 second isometric hold. Three rounds.

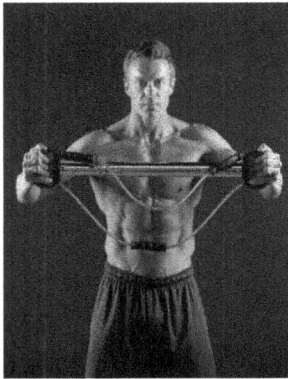
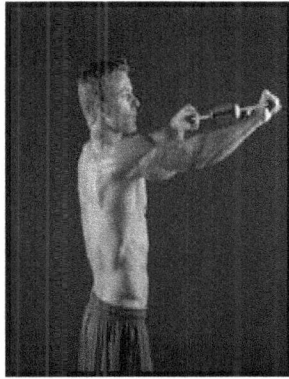
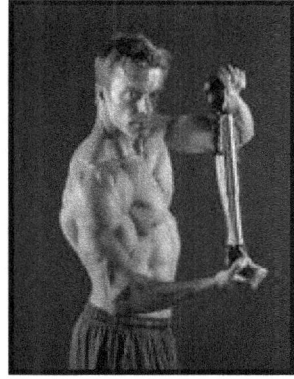

MON, WED, FRI

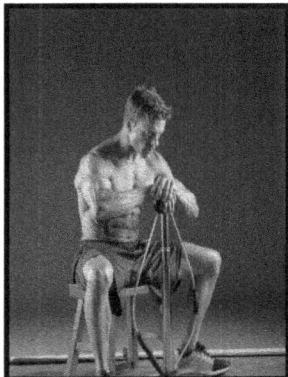
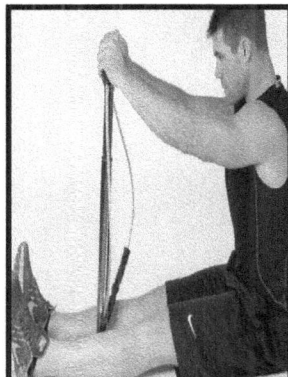
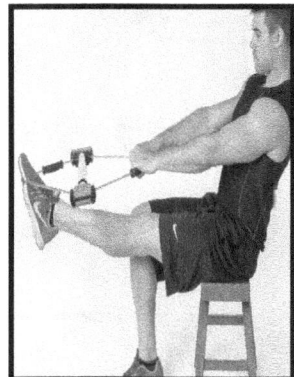

02 MAX SURGE PROGRAM

Perform all exercises non-stop. Perform 7-9 reps per bodypart, on the 9th rep perform a 10 second isometric hold. Three rounds.

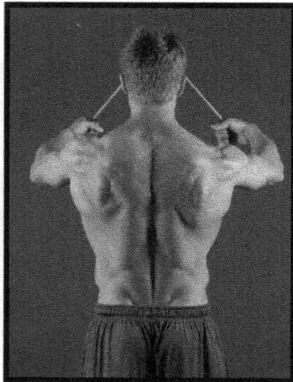

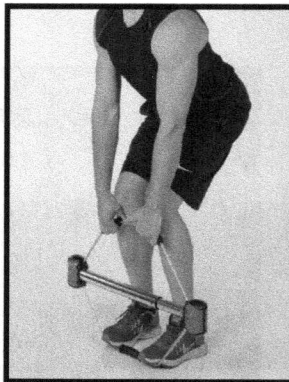

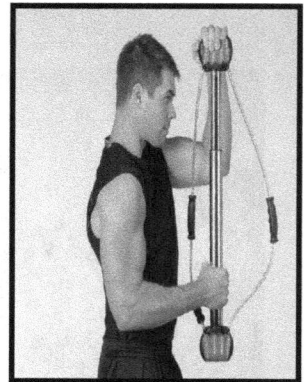

TUES, THURS, SAT

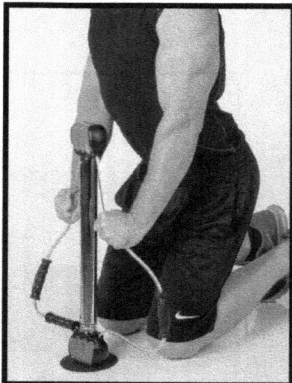

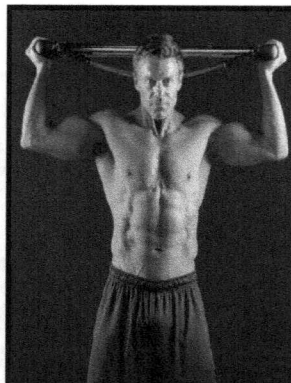

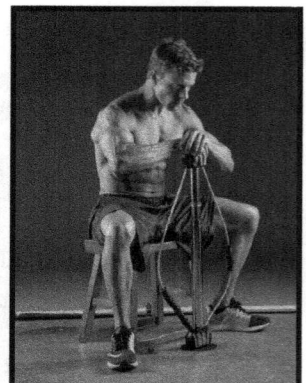

CHAPTER 2
MAX SURGE
PHASE FOUR
4 WEEKS
REP SPEED CONTRACT 2 SECONDS, RELEASE 2 SECONDS

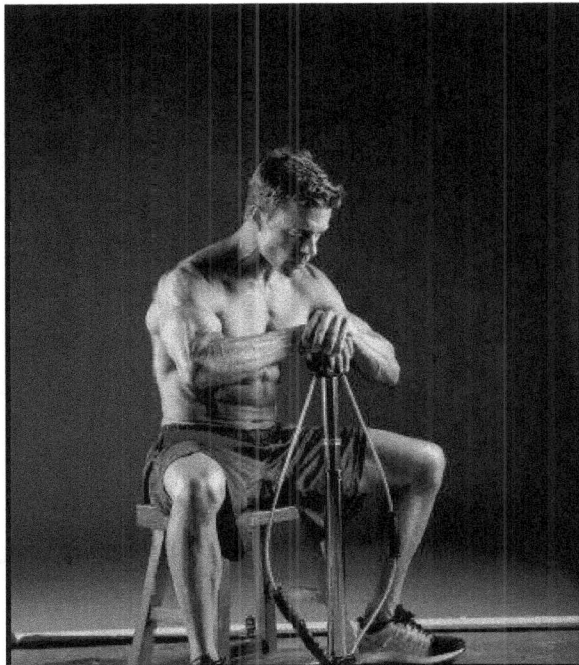

02 MAX SURGE PROGRAM

Perform 5 full reps, followed by 7 half reps. At the start position to the mid-point of the exercise stroke. On the 7th half rep perform a 7 second Isometric contraction. Three sets each exercise. All exercises are done non stop until one round is finished. Three rounds, rest 5 seconds between rounds.

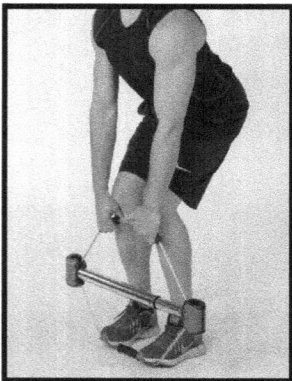 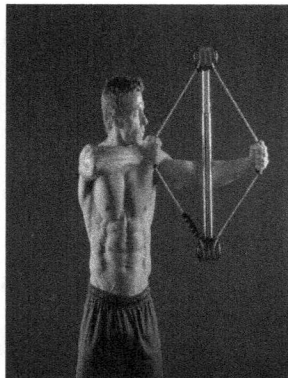 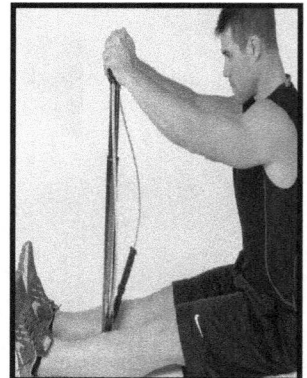

MON, WED, FRI

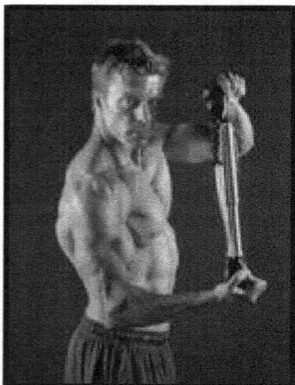 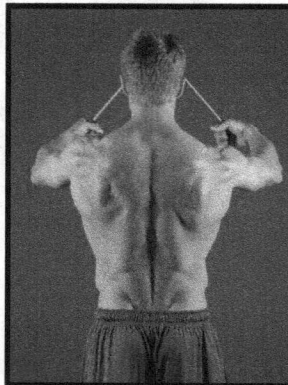 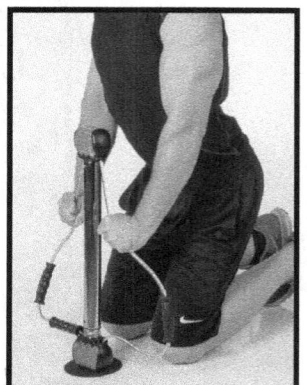

02 MAX SURGE PROGRAM

Perform 5 full reps, followed by 7 half reps. At the start position to the mid-point of the exercise stroke. On the 7th half rep perform a 7 second Isometric contraction. Three sets each exercise. All exercises are done non stop until one round is finished. Three rounds, rest 5 seconds between rounds.

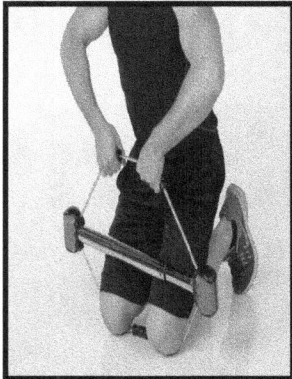

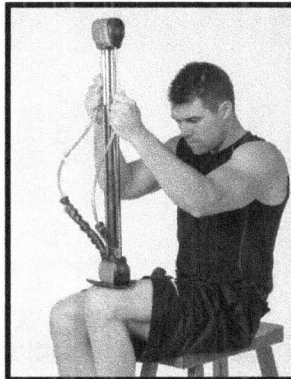

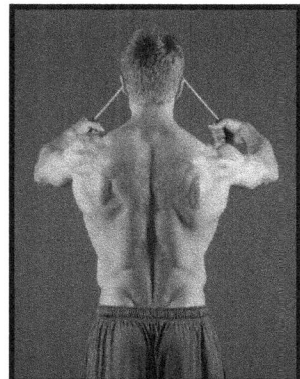

TUES, THURS, SAT

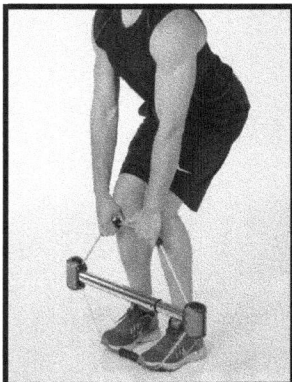

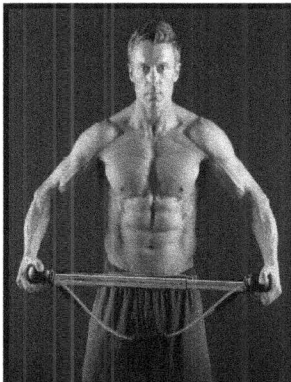

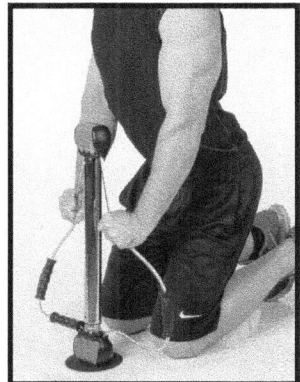

CHAPTER 3
SUPERCOMPENSATION
POWER X6 PHASE FIVE
4 WEEKS
REP SPEED CONTRACT 2 SECONDS, RELEASE 2 SECONDS

03 POWER X6 PROGRAM

Perform a 5 second Isometric contraction, followed by 15 reps. On the 15th rep perform 10 half reps from the start position to mid-point then hold for a 5 second contraction. Perform all exercises non-stop until one full round is completed. Rest 5 seconds and complete 2-3 rounds.

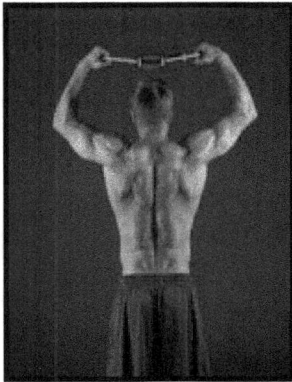 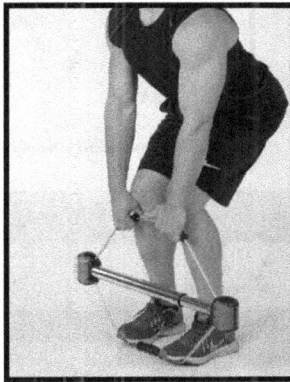 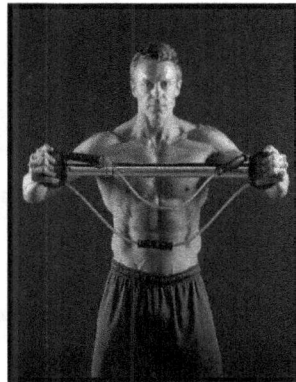

MON, WED, FRI

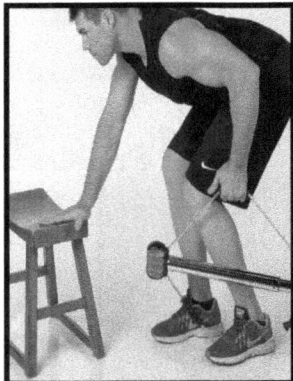 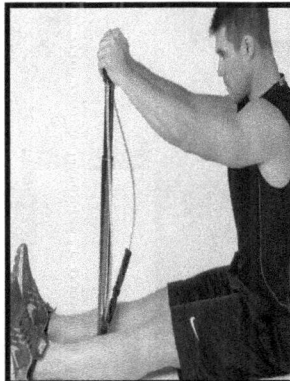 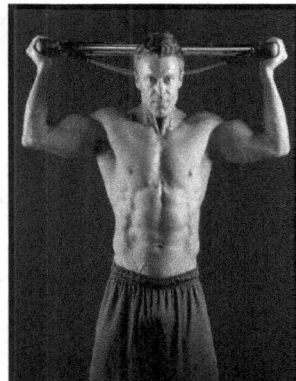

03 POWER X6 PROGRAM

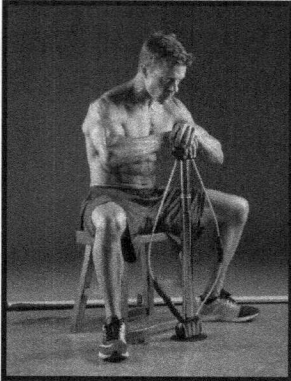

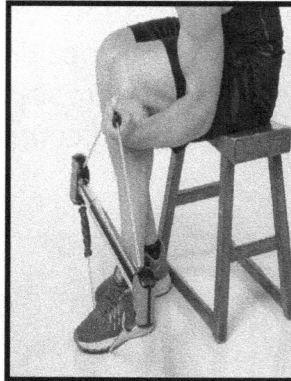

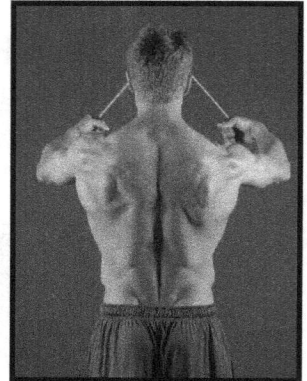

TUES, THURS, SAT

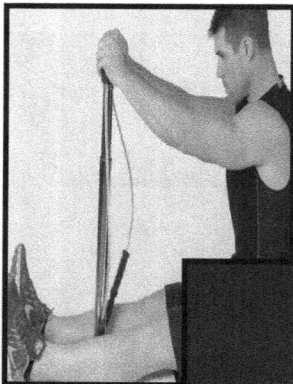

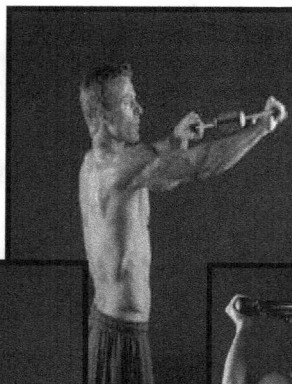

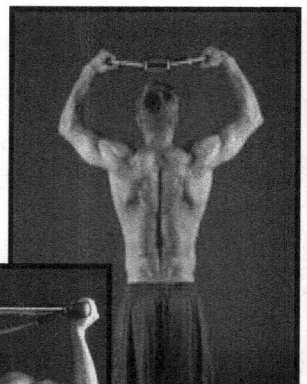

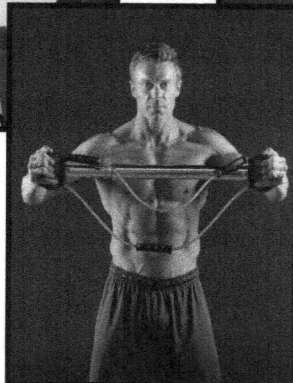

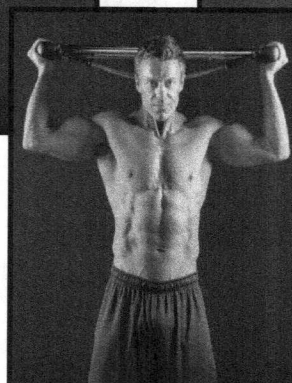

CHAPTER 3
SUPERCOMPENSATION
POWER X6 PHASE SIX
4 WEEKS
REP SPEED CONTRACT 2 SECONDS, RELEASE 2 SECONDS

03 SUPERCOMPENSATION X6 PROGRAM

Perform a 30 second Isometric contraction, followed by 10 reps. On the 10th rep perform 10 half reps from the start position to mid-point then hold for a 5 second contraction. Perform all exercises non-stop until one full round is completed. Rest 5 seconds and complete 1-2 rounds.

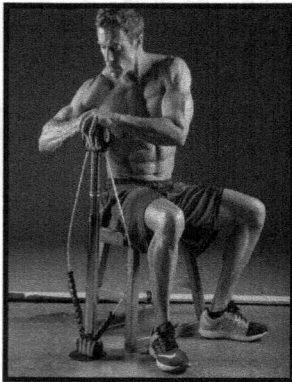 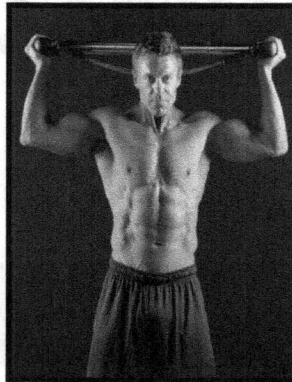 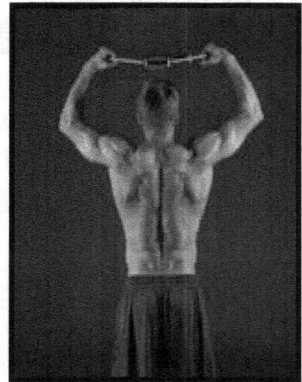

MON, WED, FRI

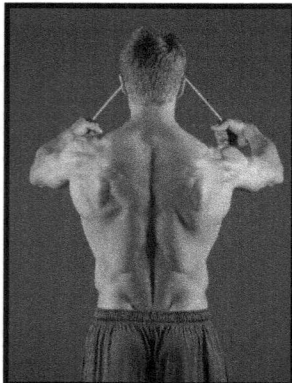 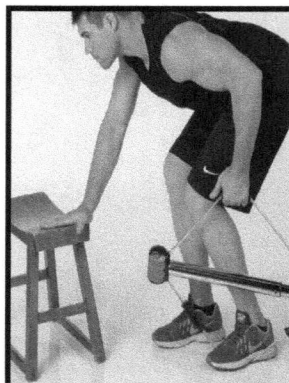 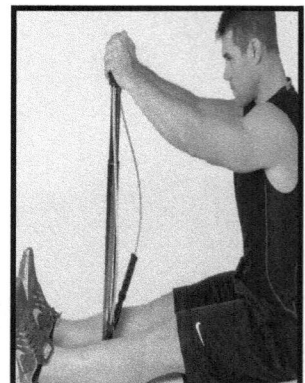

03 SUPERCOMPENSATION X6 PROGRAM

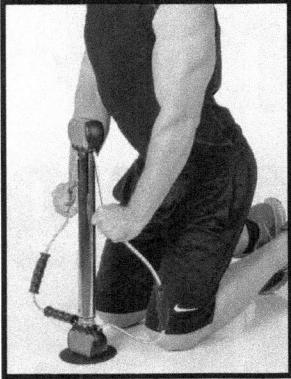

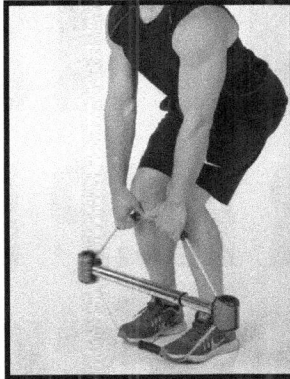

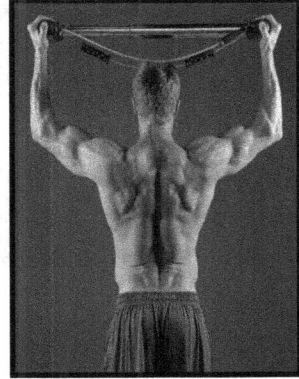

TUES, THURS, SAT

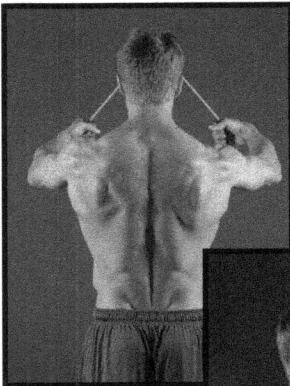

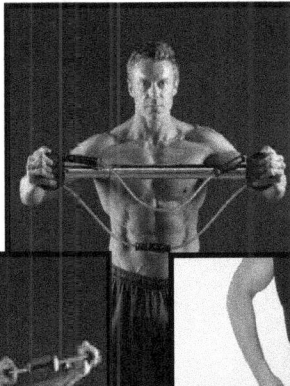

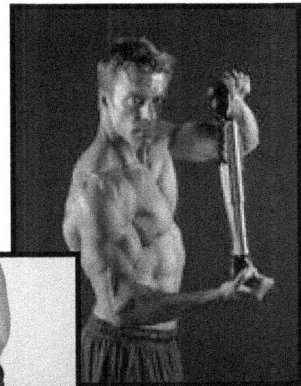

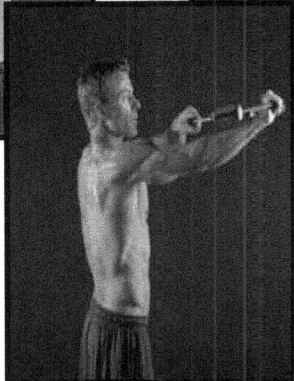

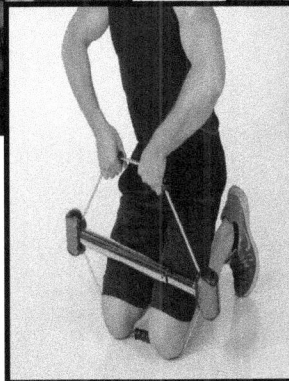

CHAPTER 4
POWER REP MAX X9
PHASE SEVEN
4 WEEKS
REP SPEED CONTRACT 2 SECONDS, RELEASE 2 SECONDS

04 POWER REP MAX X9 PROGRAM

On each exercise perform 20,10,5 reps. At the end of each rep range perform a 7 second isometric contraction. Continue until all bodyparts are completed. Perform 3 rounds in total.

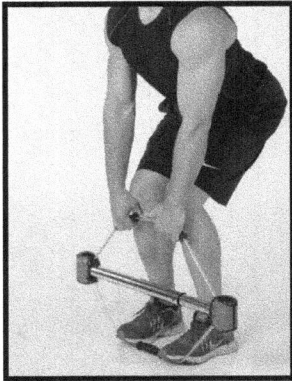
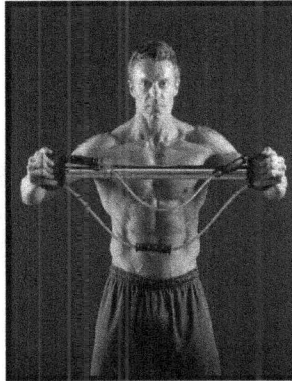
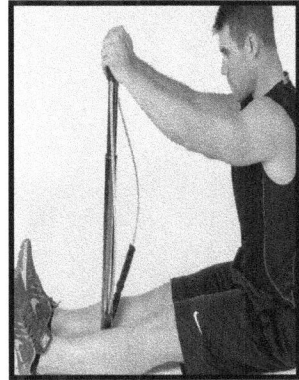

MON, WED, FRI

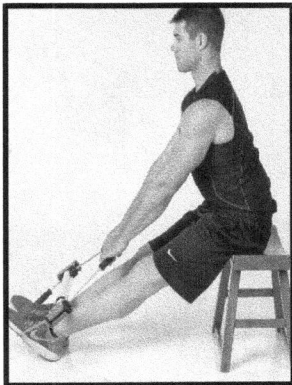
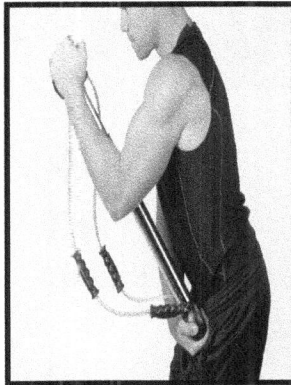
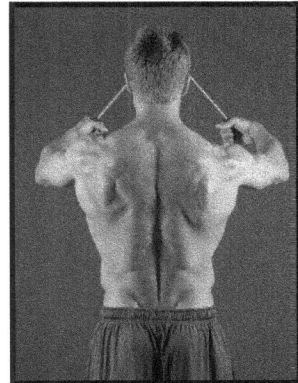

04 POWER REP MAX X9 PROGRAM

On each exercise perform 20,10,5 reps. At the end of each rep range perform a 7 second isometric contraction. Continue until all bodyparts are completed. Perform 3 rounds in total.

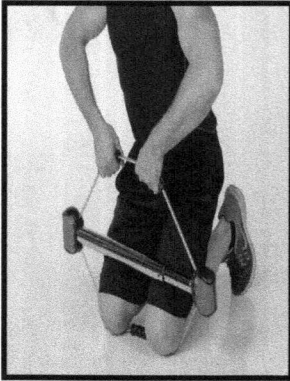

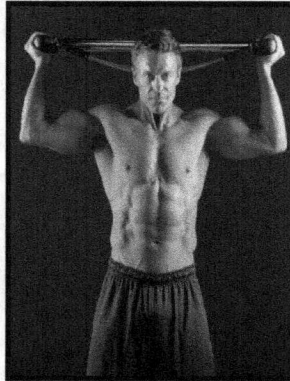

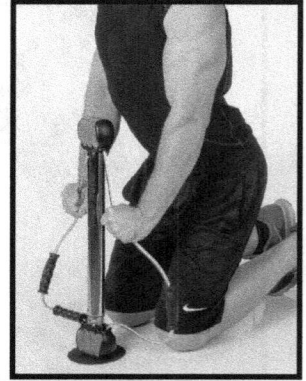

TUES, THURS, SAT

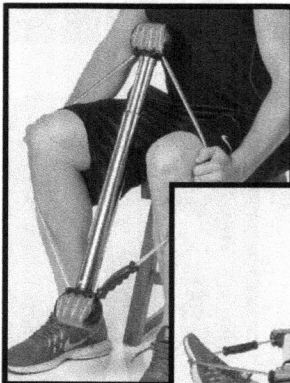

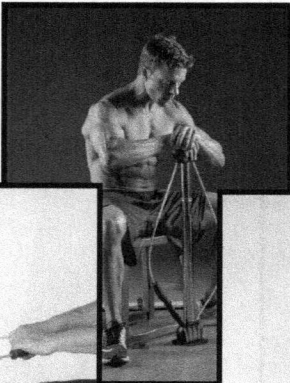

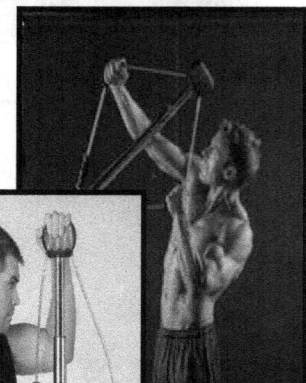

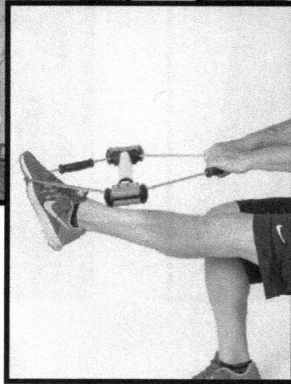

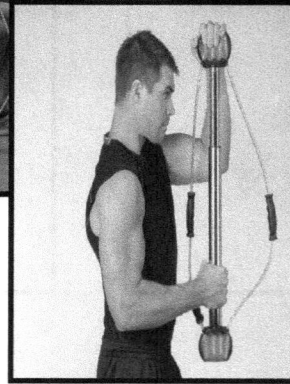

CHAPTER 5
POWER PUMP 30
PHASE EIGHT
4 WEEKS
REP SPEED CONTRACT 2 SECONDS, RELEASE 2 SECONDS

POWER PUMP 30 PROGRAM

05 POWER PUMP 30 PROGRAM DAY ONE

HOW TO PERFORM THIS ROUTINE: Perform 30 reps, followed by an isometric contraction for 30 seconds. **PERFORM 1-2 ROUNDS (SETS)**

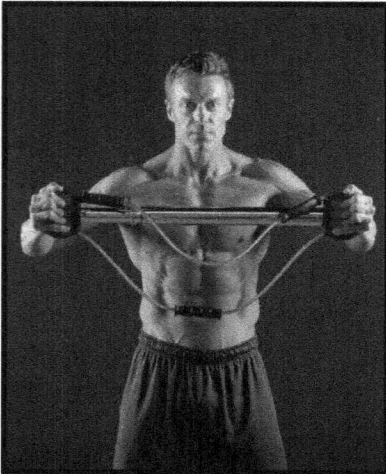

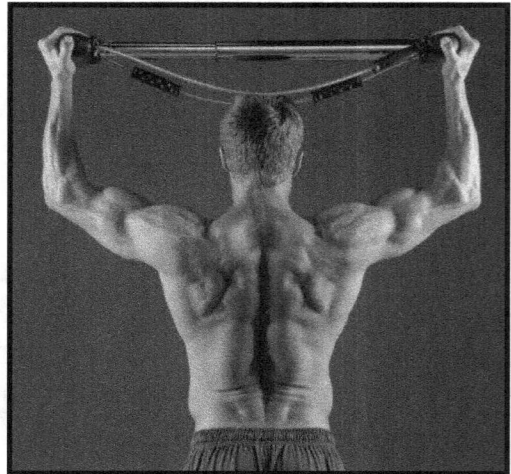

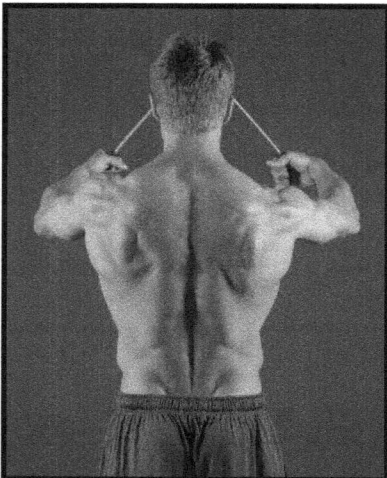

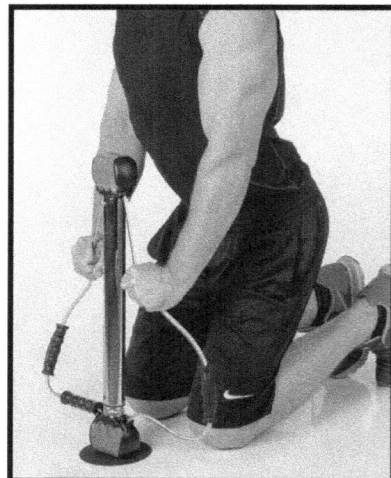

POWER PUMP 30 PROGRAM

05 POWER PUMP 30 PROGRAM DAY TWO

HOW TO PERFORM THIS ROUTINE: Perform 30 reps, followed by an isometric contraction for 30 seconds. **PERFORM 1-2 ROUNDS (SETS)**

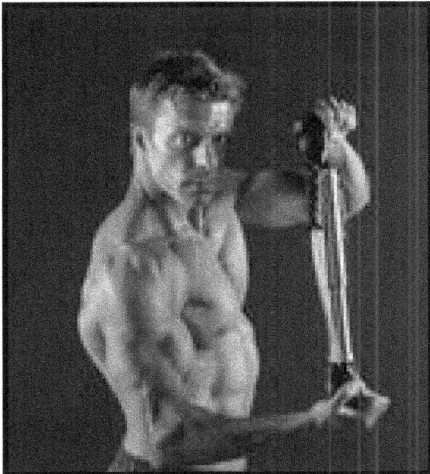

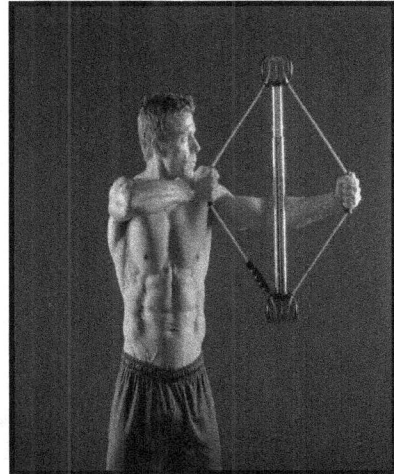

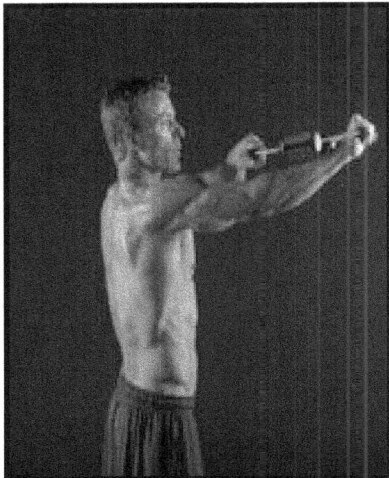

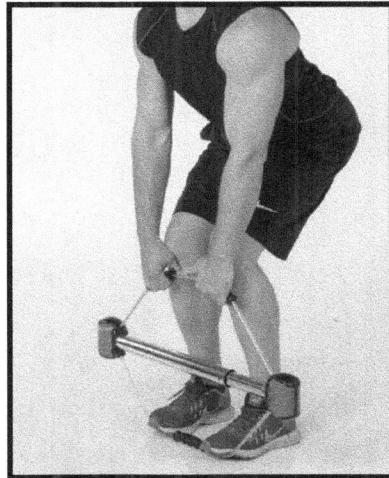

POWER PUMP 30 PROGRAM

05 POWER PUMP 30 DAY THREE

HOW TO PERFORM THIS ROUTINE: Perform 30 reps, followed by an isometric contraction for 30 seconds. **PERFORM 1-2 ROUNDS (SETS)**

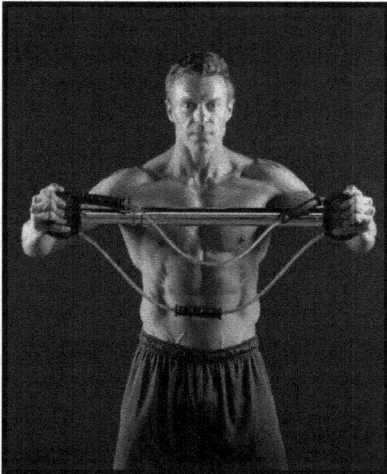

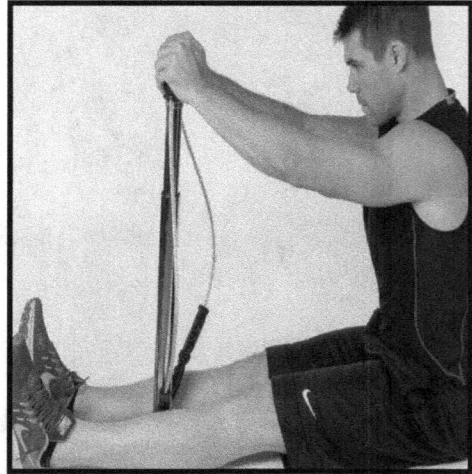

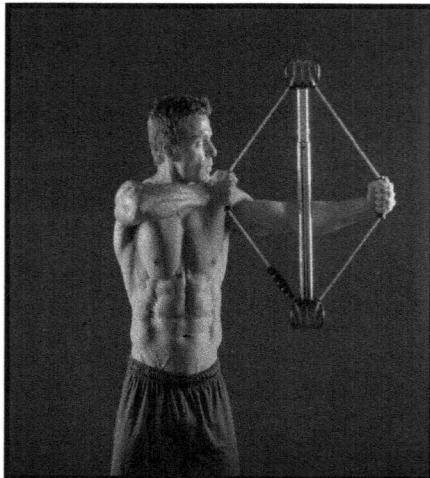

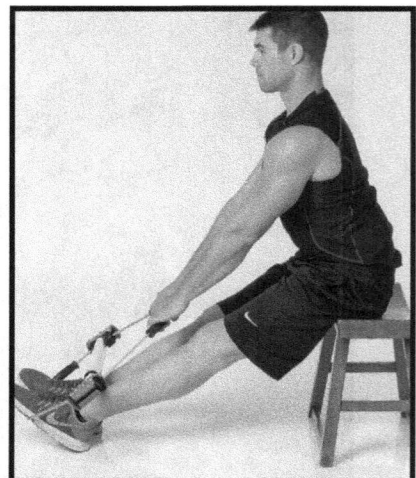

POWER PUMP 30 PROGRAM

05 POWER PUMP 30 DAY FOUR

HOW TO PERFORM THIS ROUTINE: Perform 30 reps, followed by an isometric contraction for 30 seconds. **PERFORM 1-2 ROUNDS (SETS)**

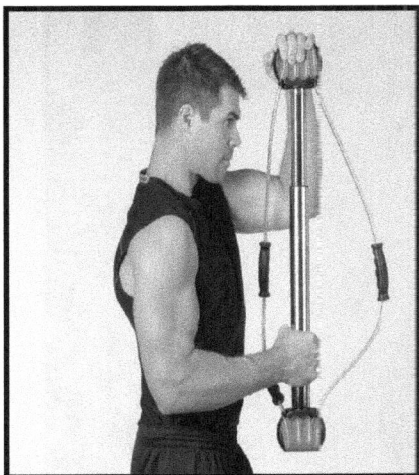

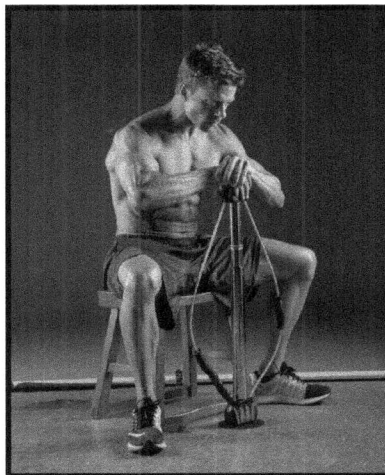

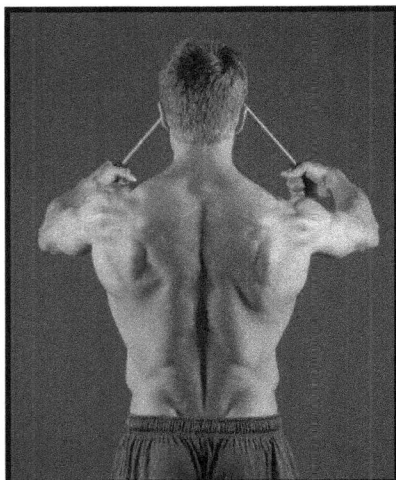

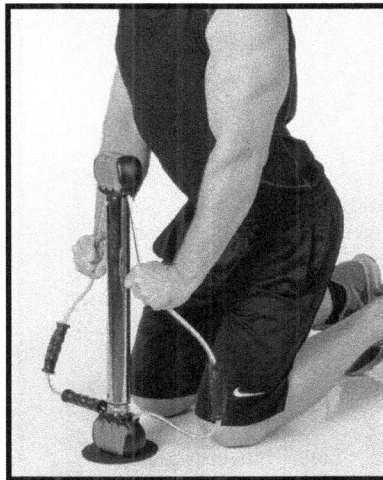

POWER PUMP 30 PROGRAM

05 POWER PUMP 30 DAY FIVE

HOW TO PERFORM THIS ROUTINE: Perform 30 reps, followed by an isometric contraction for 30 seconds. **PERFORM 1-2 ROUNDS (SETS)**

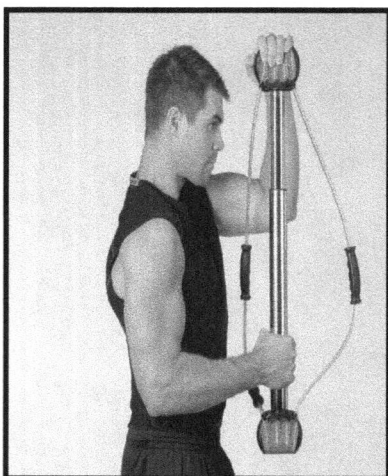

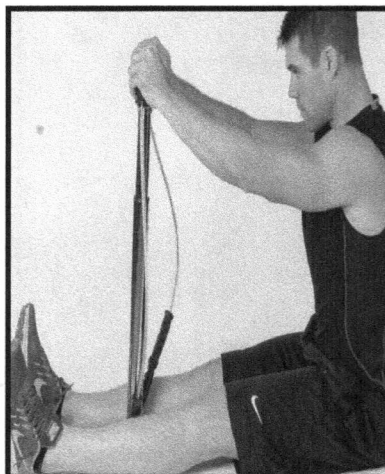

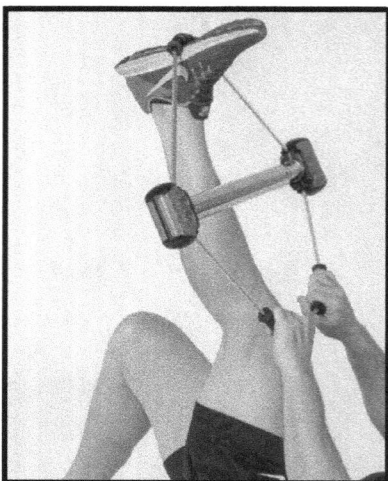

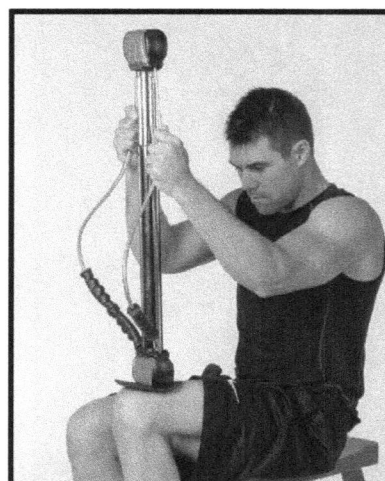

POWER X-PUMP PROGRAM

06 POWER X-PUMP PROGRAM

MONDAY, WEDNESDAY, FRIDAY
HOW TO PERFORM THIS ROUTINE: You contract for 2 seconds and release for a slow 6 seconds. Perform 3 reps; each rep perform an isometric contraction for 1 second. Perform 2-3 rounds. Perform all exercises then rest 20 seconds and repeat. **Perform plan for 4 weeks before moving to Phase Ten.**

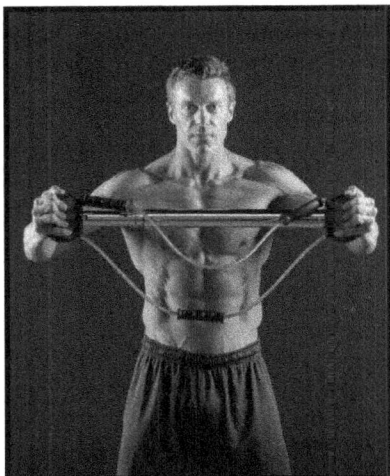

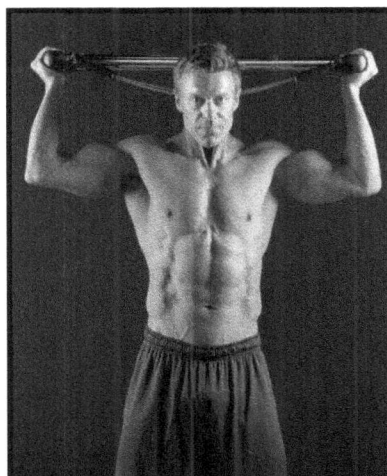

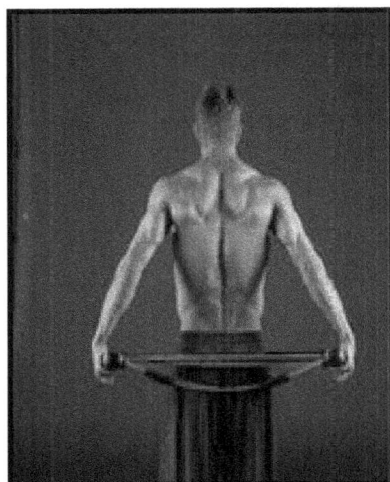

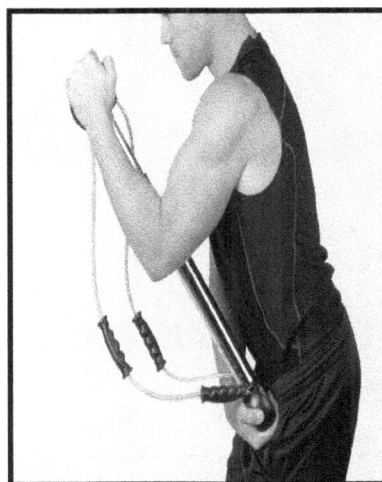

POWER X-PUMP PROGRAM

06 POWER X-PUMP PROGRAM

MONDAY,WEDNESDAY,FRIDAY
Routine continued.............

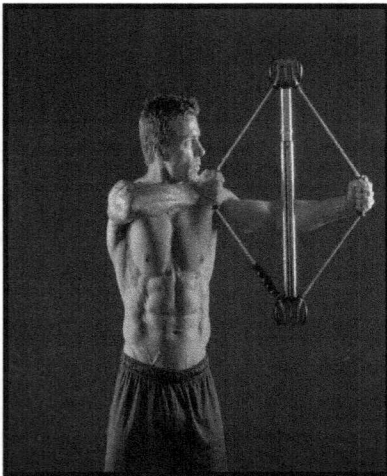

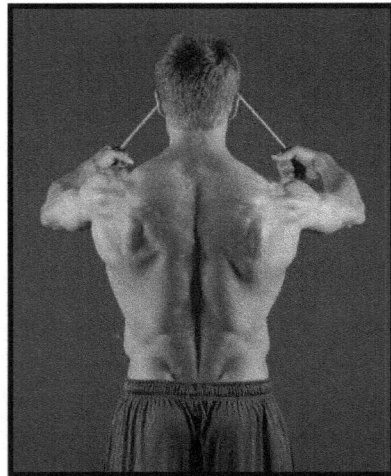

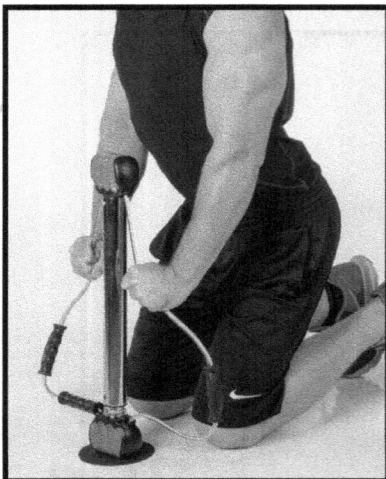

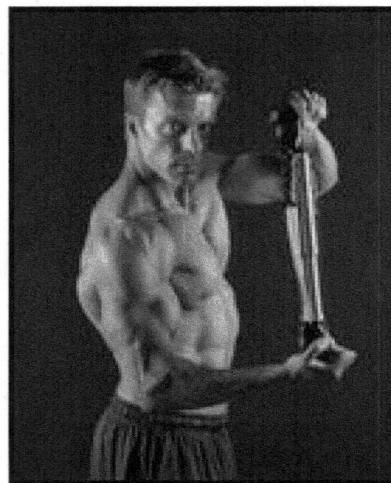

POWER X-PUMP PROGRAM

06 POWER X-PUMP PROGRAM

MONDAY, WEDNESDAY, FRIDAY
Routine continued............

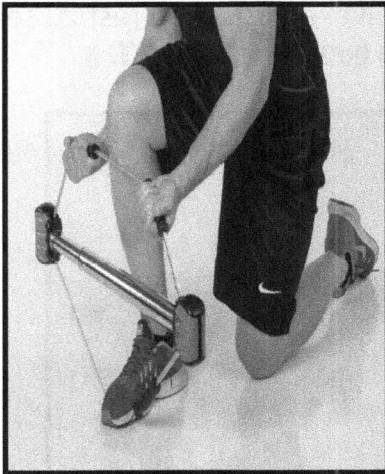

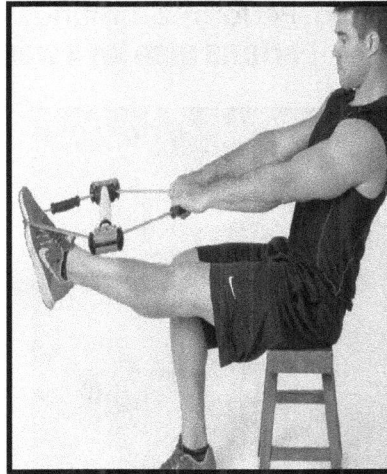

PHASE NINE MON, WED, FRI

POWER X-PUMP PROGRAM

06 POWER X-PUMP PROGRAM

TUESDAY, THURSDAY, SATURDAY
HOW TO PERFORM THIS ROUTINE: You contract for 2 seconds and release for a slow 6 seconds. Perform 3 reps; each rep perform an isometric contraction for 1 second. Perform 2-3 rounds. Perform all exercises then rest 20 seconds and repeat. **Perform plan for 4 weeks before moving to Phase Ten.**

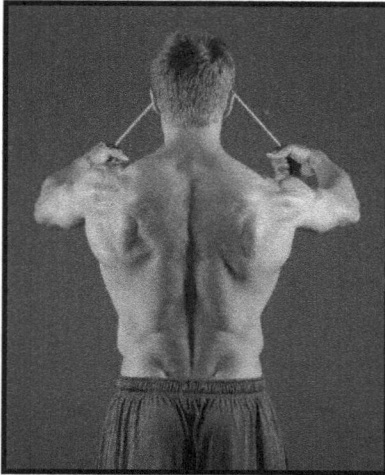

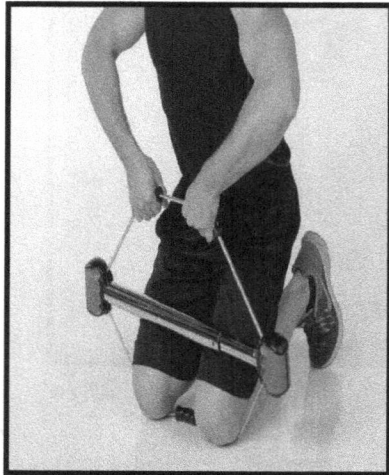

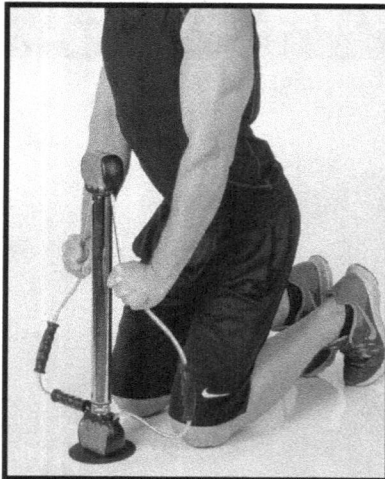

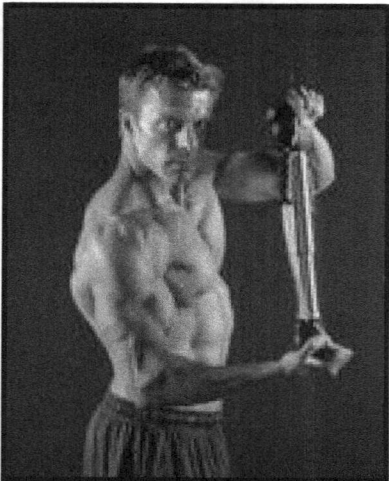

POWER X-PUMP PROGRAM

06 POWER X-PUMP PROGRAM

TUESDAY, THURSDAY, SATURDAY
Routine continued....................

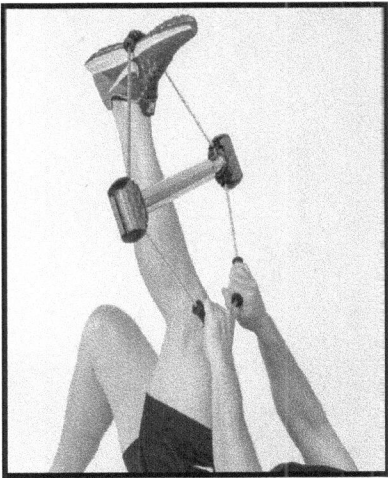

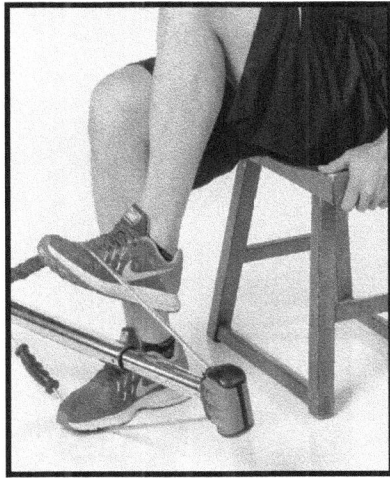

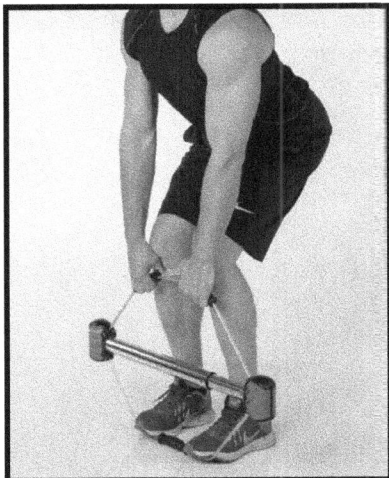

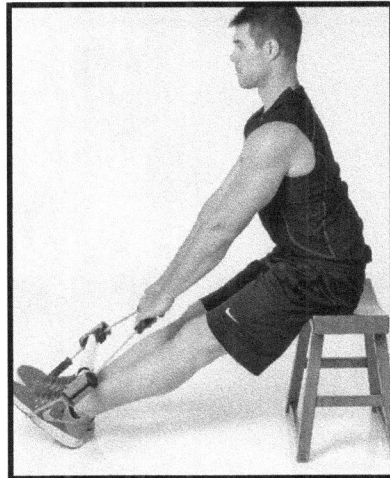

POWER X-PUMP PROGRAM

06 POWER X-PUMP PROGRAM

TUESDAY, THURSDAY, SATURDAY
Routine continued....................

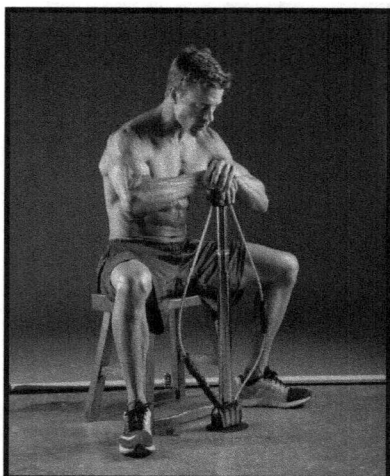

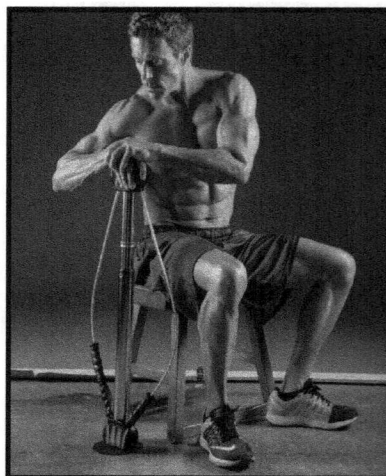

PHASE NINE TUES, THURS, SAT.

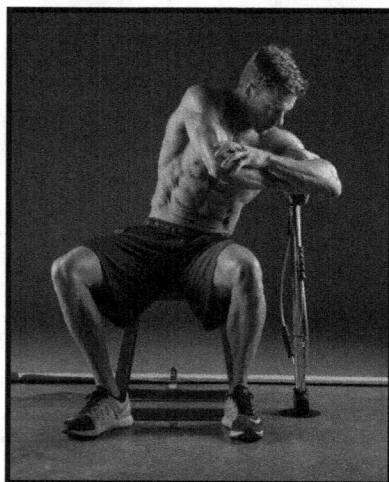

DENSITY REP RANGE X2

07 DENSITY REP RANGE X2 PROGRAM 25,15,5

MONDAY, WEDNESDAY, FRIDAY
HOW TO PERFORM THIS ROUTINE: Contract 2 seconds release 3 seconds. Perform 25 reps followed by a 1 second isometric, 15 reps followed by another 1 second isometric, then a final 5 reps. On the 5th rep hold for a 30 second Isometric contraction. One round only. **Perform program for 4 weeks**

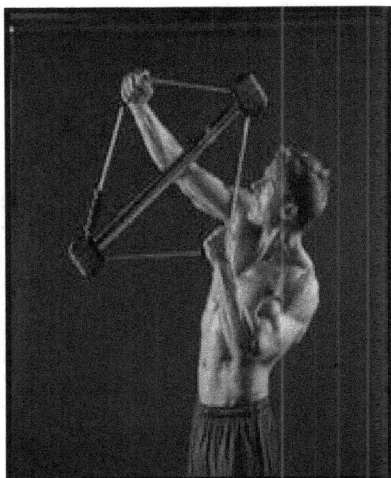

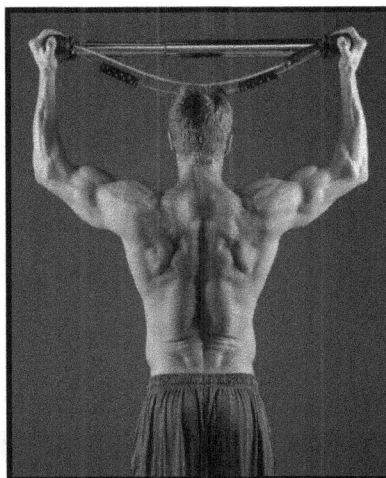

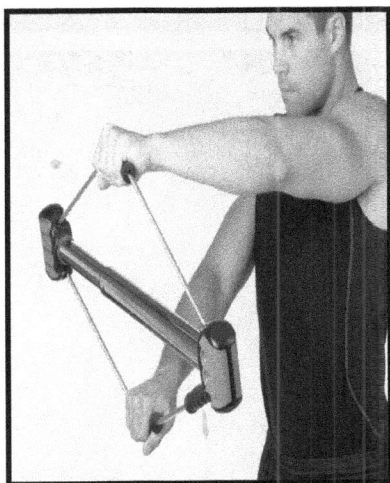

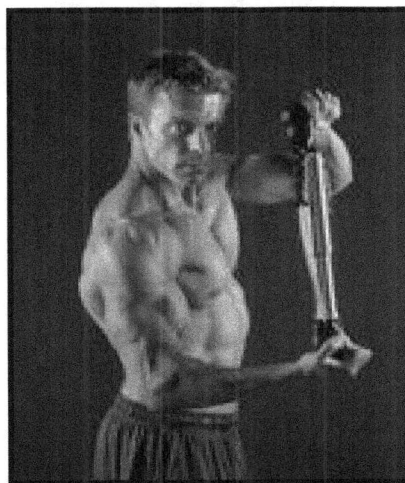

DENSITY REP RANGE X2

07 DENSITY REP RANGE X2 PROGRAM 25,15,5

MONDAY, WEDNESDAY, FRIDAY
Routine continued............

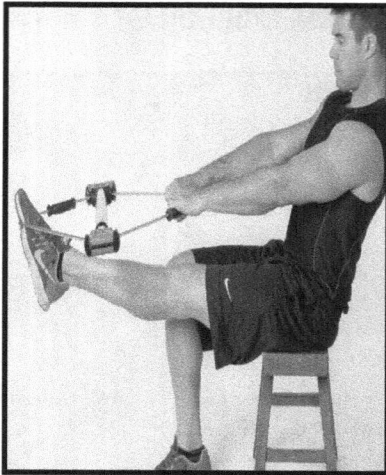

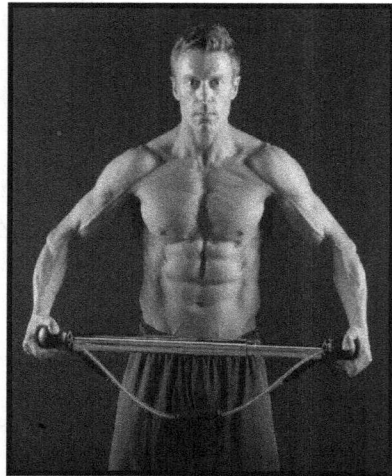

PHASE TEN   MON, WED, FRI.

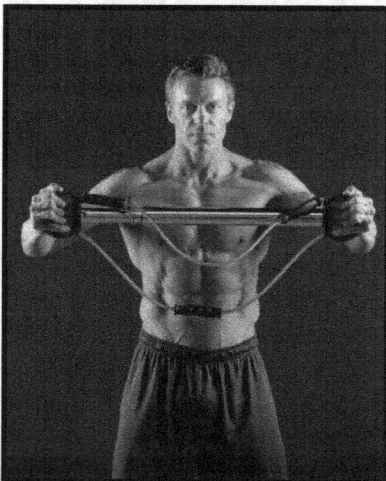

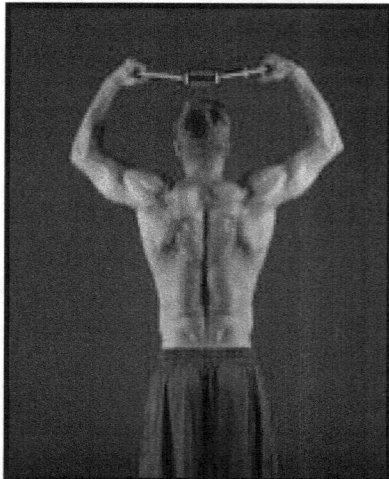

DENSITY REP RANGE X2

07 DENSITY REP RANGE X2 PROGRAM 25,15,5

TUESDAY, THURSDAY, SATURDAY
HOW TO PERFORM THIS ROUTINE: Contract 2 seconds release 3 seconds. Perform 25 reps followed by a 1 second isometric, 15 reps followed by another 1 second isometric, then a final 5 reps. On the 5th rep hold for a 30 second Isometric contraction. One round only. **Perform program for 4 weeks**

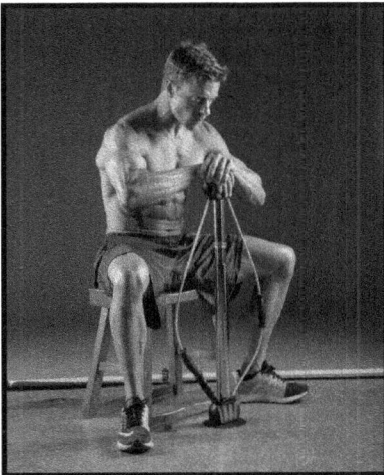

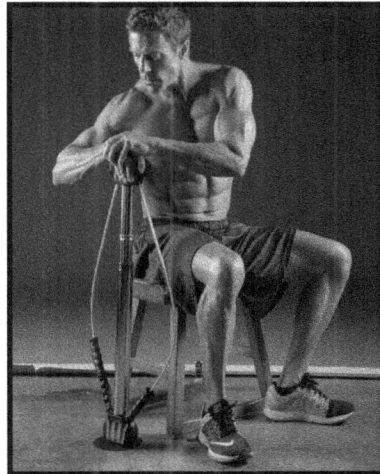

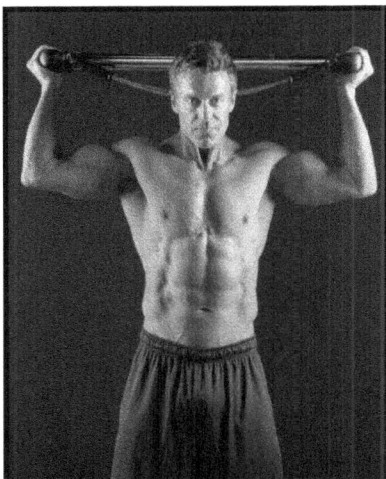

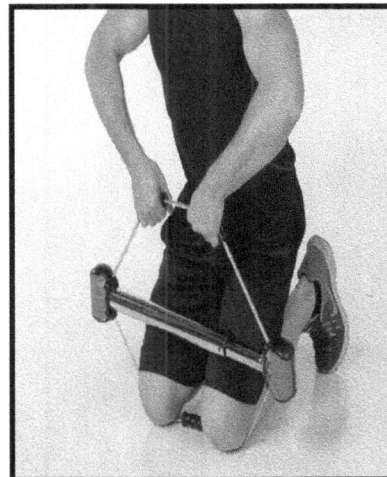

DENSITY REP RANGE X2

07 DENSITY REP RANGE X2 PROGRAM 25,15,5

TUESDAY, THURSDAY, SATURDAY
Routine continued...................

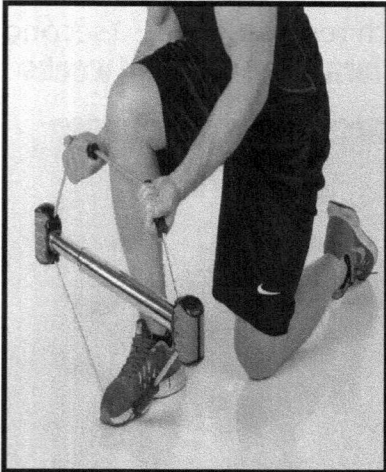

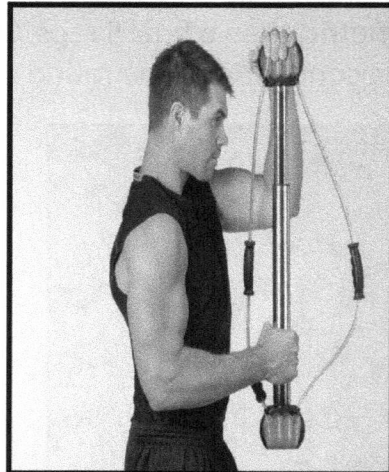

PHASE TEN   TUES, THURS, SAT.

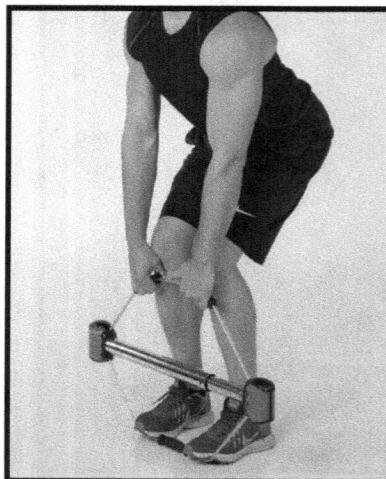

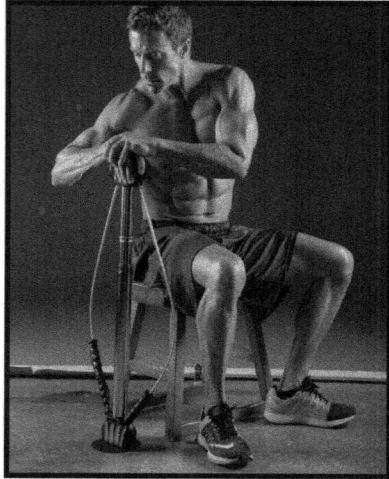

CHAPTER 8
DENSITY REP RANGE X4
PHASE 11
4 WEEKS

REP SPEED CONTRACT 2 SECONDS, RELEASE 2 SECONDS
1ST WEEK 30 REPS, 10 SECOND ISOMETRIC... 2-3 ROUNDS
2ND WEEK 7-9 REPS, 20 SECOND ISOMETRIC.. 3 ROUNDS
3RD WEEK 10 REPS, 20 SECOND ISOMETRIC... 3 ROUNDS
4TH WEEK 20 REPS, 15 SECONDS ISOMETRIC..... 3 ROUNDS

REP RANGE X4

08 DENSITY REP RANGE X4

HOW TO PERFORM THIS ROUTINE:
1ST Week: 30 reps, 10 second Isometric contraction 2-3 rounds.
2ND Week: 7-9 reps, 20 second Isometric contraction 3 rounds.
3RD Week: 10 reps, 30 second Isometric contraction 3 rounds.
4th Week: 20 reps, 15 second Isometric contraction 3 rounds.

DAY ONE

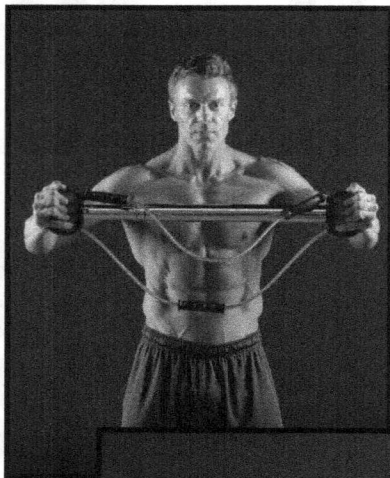

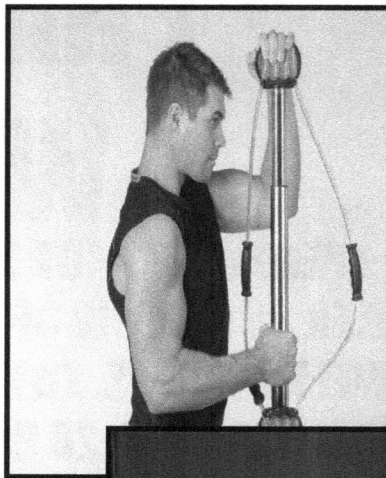

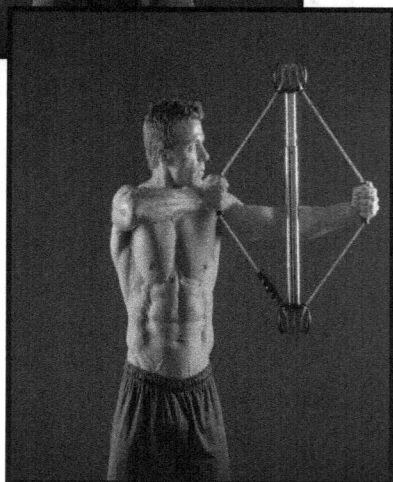

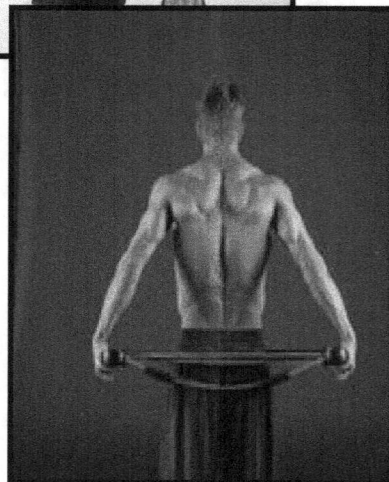

REP RANGE X4

08 DENSITY REP RANGE X4

HOW TO PERFORM THIS ROUTINE:
1ST Week: 30 reps, 10 second Isometric contraction 2-3 rounds.
2ND Week: 7-9 reps, 20 second Isometric contraction 3 rounds.
3RD Week: 10 reps, 30 second Isometric contraction 3 rounds.
4th Week: 20 reps, 15 second Isometric contraction 3 rounds.

DAY ONE continued.........

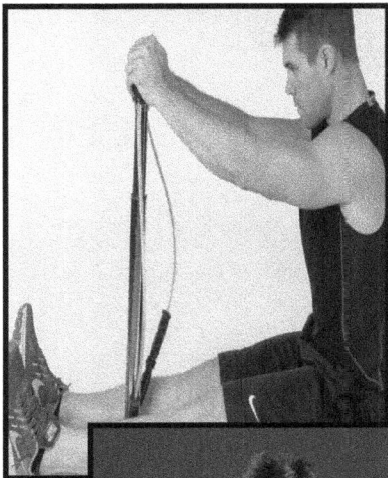

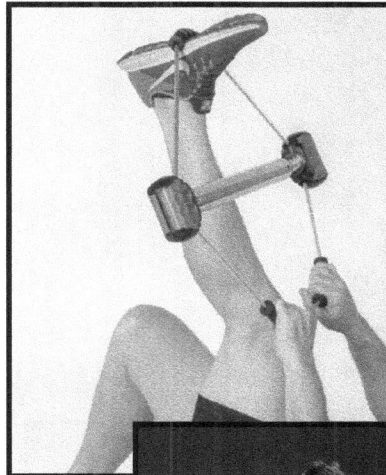

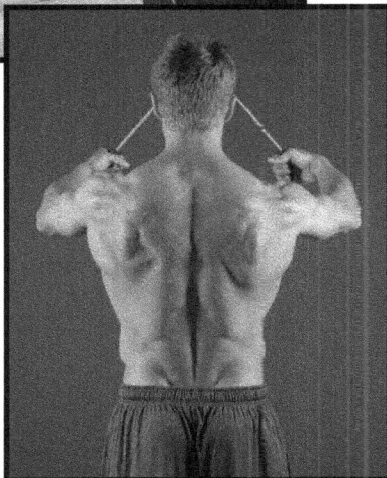

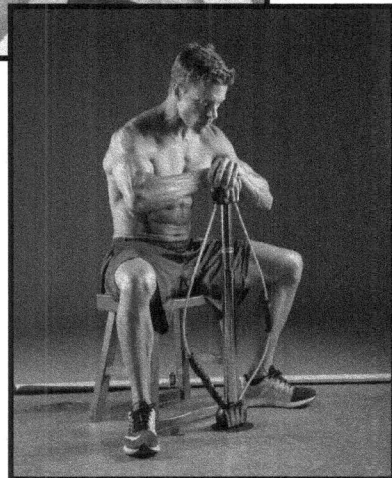

REP RANGE X4

08 DENSITY REP RANGE X4

HOW TO PERFORM THIS ROUTINE:

1ST Week: 30 reps, 10 second Isometric contraction 2-3 rounds.
2ND Week: 7-9 reps, 20 second Isometric contraction 3 rounds.
3RD Week: 10 reps, 30 second Isometric contraction 3 rounds.
4th Week: 20 reps, 15 second Isometric contraction 3 rounds.

DAY TWO

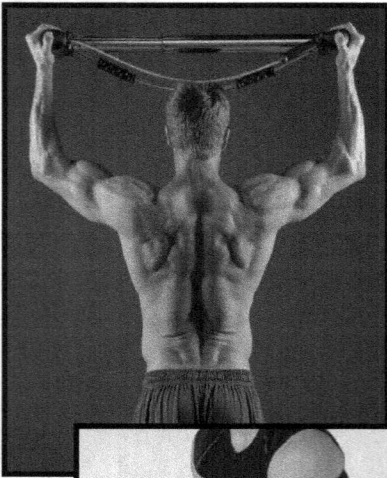
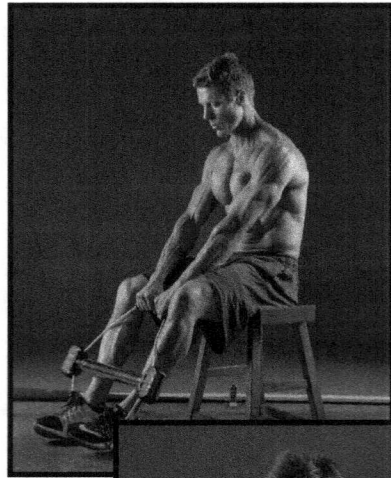
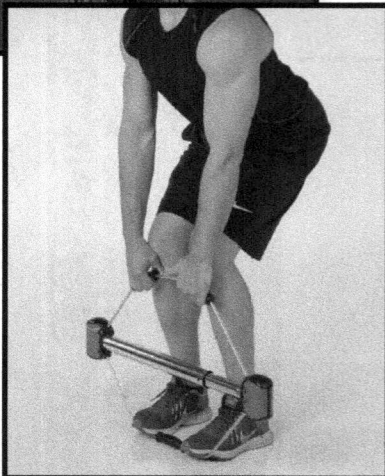
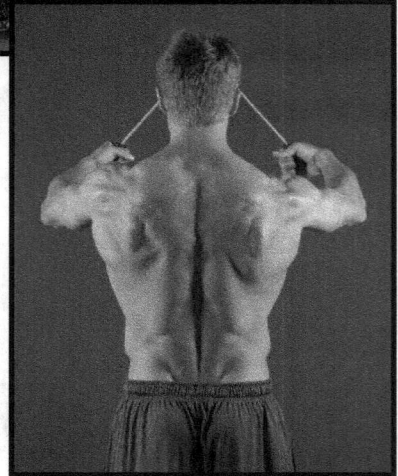

REP RANGE X4

08 REP RANGE X4

HOW TO PERFORM THIS ROUTINE:
1ST Week: 30 reps, 10 second Isometric contraction 2-3 rounds.
2ND Week: 7-9 reps, 20 second Isometric contraction 3 rounds.
3RD Week: 10 reps, 30 second Isometric contraction 3 rounds.
4th Week: 20 reps, 15 second Isometric contraction 3 rounds.

DAY TWO continued............

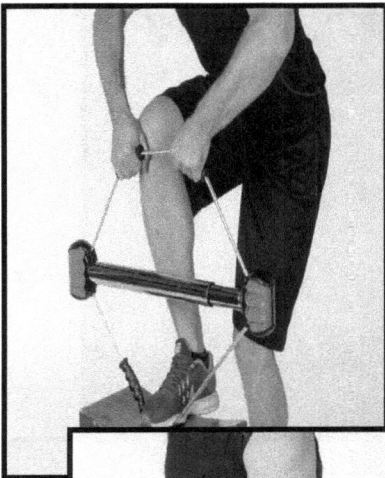
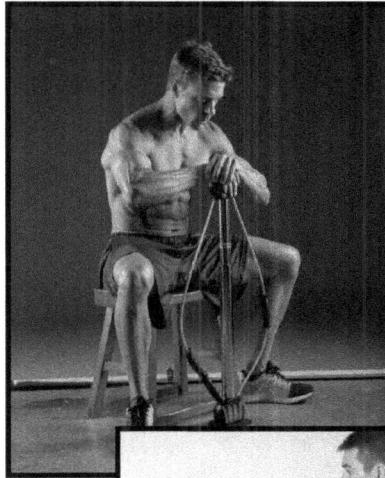
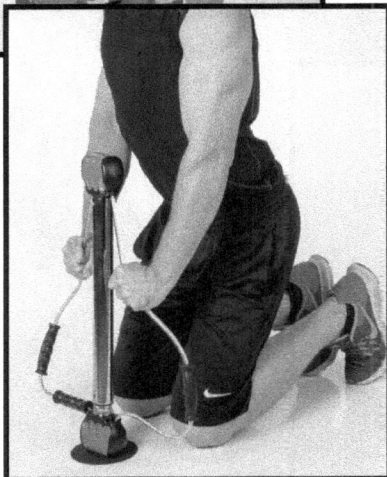
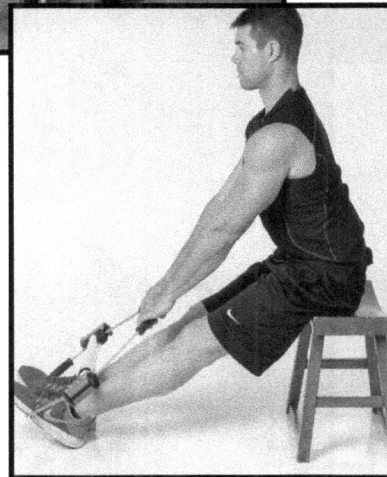

REP RANGE X4

08 REP RANGE X4

HOW TO PERFORM THIS ROUTINE:
1ST Week: 30 reps, 10 second Isometric contraction 2-3 rounds.
2ND Week: 7-9 reps, 20 second Isometric contraction 3 rounds.
3RD Week: 10 reps, 30 second Isometric contraction 3 rounds.
4th Week: 20 reps, 15 second Isometric contraction 3 rounds.

DAY THREE

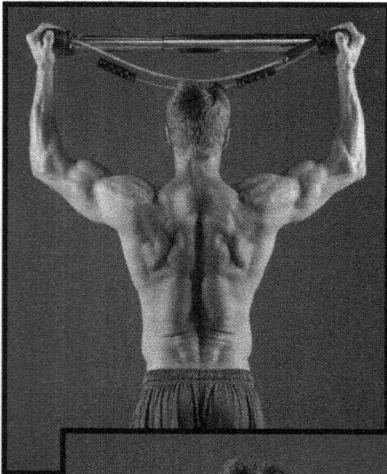

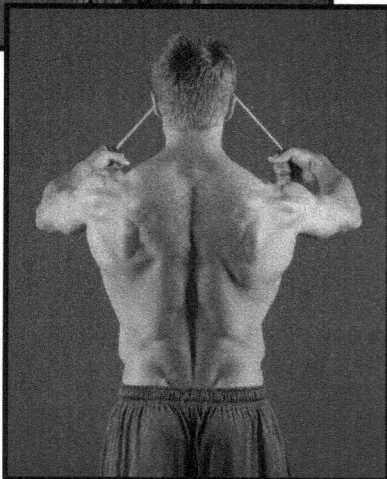

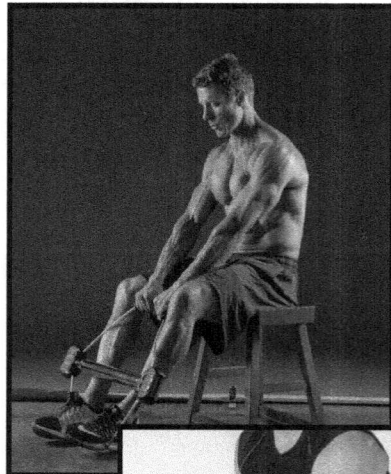

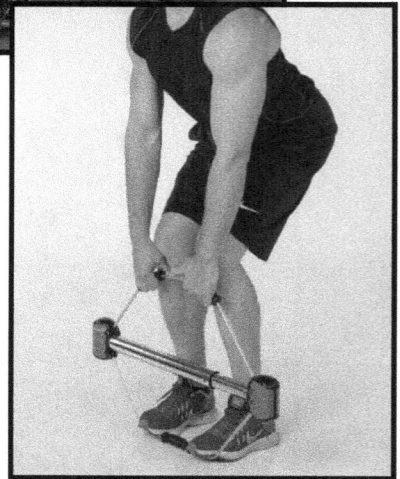

REP RANGE X4

08 REP RANGE X4

HOW TO PERFORM THIS ROUTINE:
1ST Week: 30 reps, 10 second Isometric contraction 2-3 rounds.
2ND Week: 7-9 reps, 20 second Isometric contraction 3 rounds.
3RD Week: 10 reps, 30 second Isometric contraction 3 rounds.
4th Week: 20 reps, 15 second Isometric contraction 3 rounds.

DAY THREE continued.......

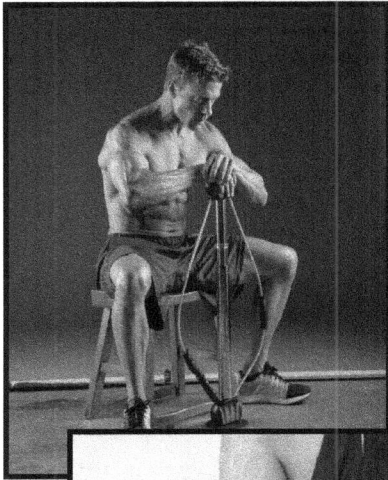

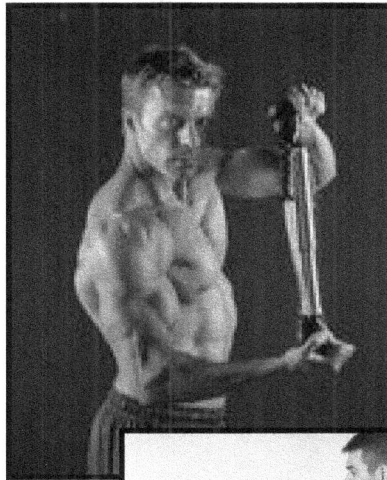

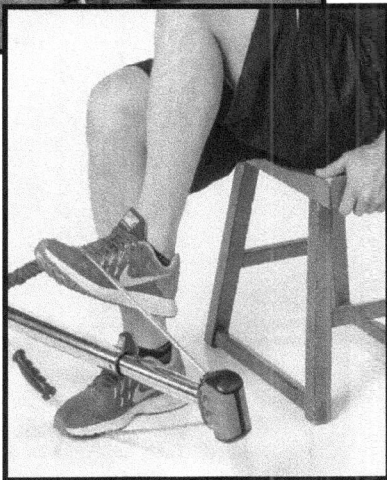

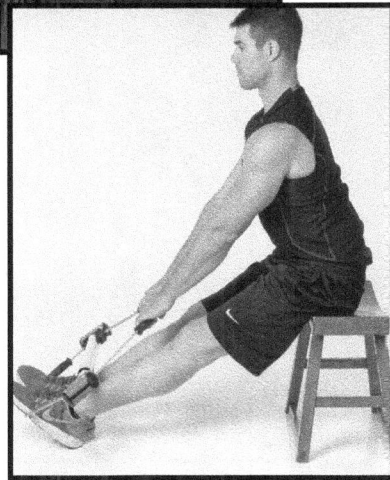

REP RANGE X4

08 REP RANGE X4

HOW TO PERFORM THIS ROUTINE:
1ST Week: 30 reps, 10 second Isometric contraction 2-3 rounds.
2ND Week: 7-9 reps, 20 second Isometric contraction 3 rounds.
3RD Week: 10 reps, 30 second Isometric contraction 3 rounds.
4th Week: 20 reps, 15 second Isometric contraction 3 rounds.

DAY THREE continued.......

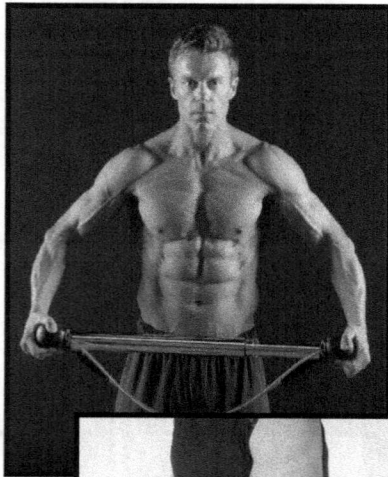

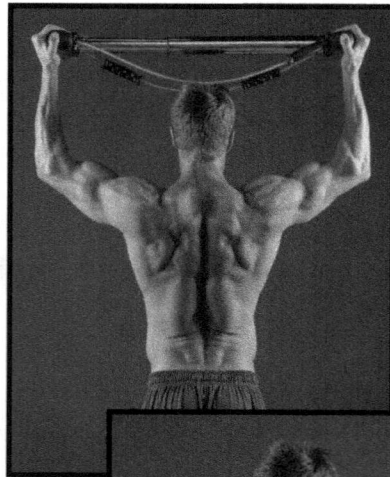

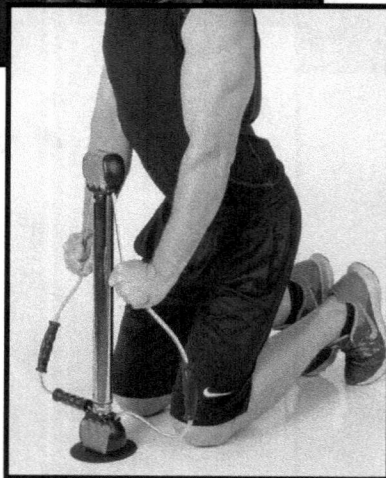

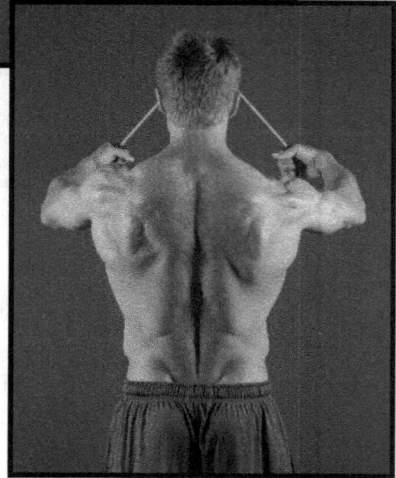

REP RANGE X4

08 REP RANGE X4

HOW TO PERFORM THIS ROUTINE:
1ST Week: 30 reps, 10 second Isometric contraction 2-3 rounds.
2ND Week: 7-9 reps, 20 second Isometric contraction 3 rounds.
3RD Week: 10 reps, 30 second Isometric contraction 3 rounds.
4th Week: 20 reps, 15 second Isometric contraction 3 rounds.

DAY FOUR

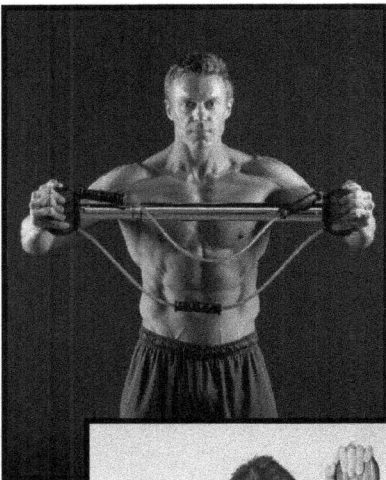
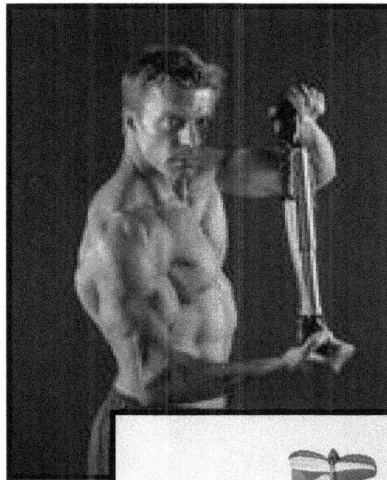
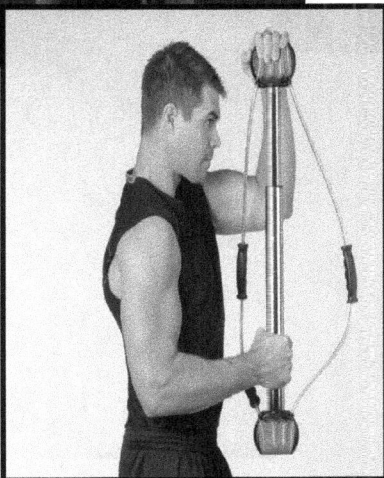
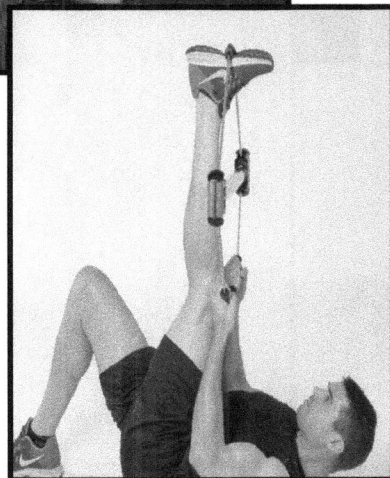

REP RANGE X4

08 REP RANGE X4

HOW TO PERFORM THIS ROUTINE:
1ST Week: 30 reps, 10 second Isometric contraction 2-3 rounds.
2ND Week: 7-9 reps, 20 second Isometric contraction 3 rounds.
3RD Week: 10 reps, 30 second Isometric contraction 3 rounds.
4th Week: 20 reps, 15 second Isometric contraction 3 rounds.

DAY FOUR continued......

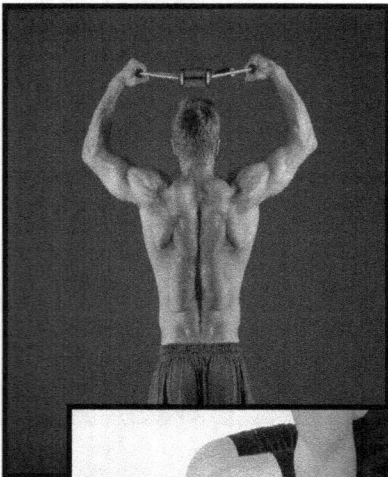

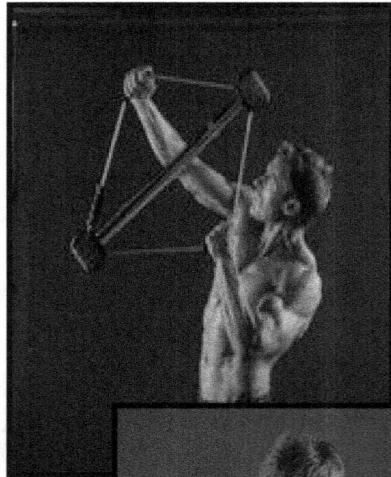

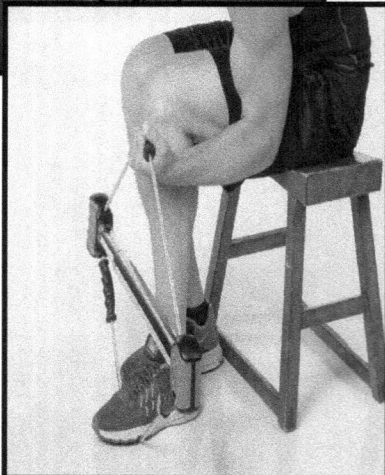

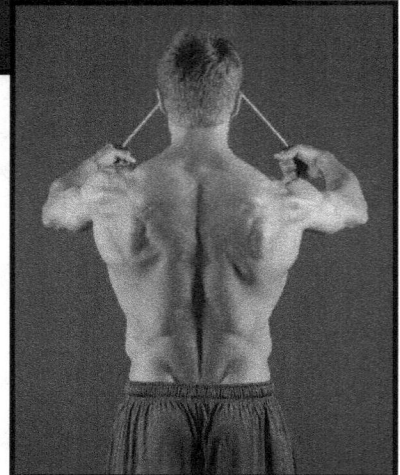

REP RANGE X4

08 REP RANGE X4

HOW TO PERFORM THIS ROUTINE:
1ST Week: 30 reps, 10 second Isometric contraction 2-3 rounds.
2ND Week: 7-9 reps, 20 second Isometric contraction 3 rounds.
3RD Week: 10 reps, 30 second Isometric contraction 3 rounds.
4th Week: 20 reps, 15 second Isometric contraction 3 rounds.

DAY FIVE

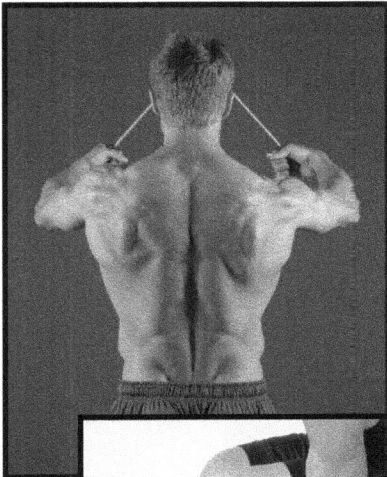
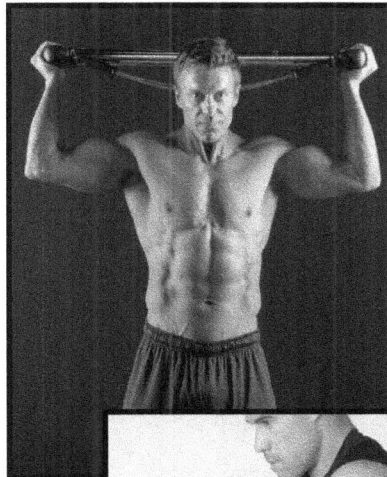
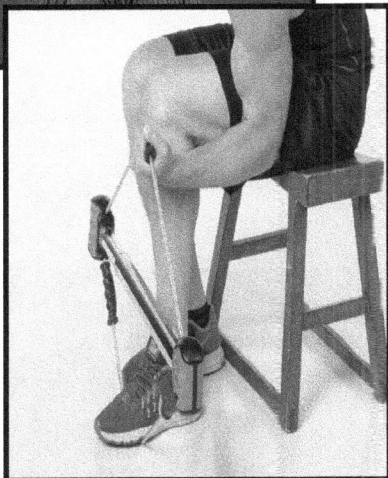
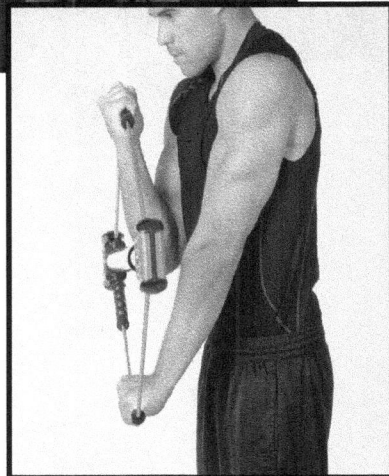

REP RANGE X4

08 REP RANGE X4

HOW TO PERFORM THIS ROUTINE:
1ST Week: 30 reps, 10 second Isometric contraction 2-3 rounds.
2ND Week: 7-9 reps, 20 second Isometric contraction 3 rounds.
3RD Week: 10 reps, 30 second Isometric contraction 3 rounds.
4th Week: 20 reps, 15 second Isometric contraction 3 rounds.

DAY FIVE continued.....

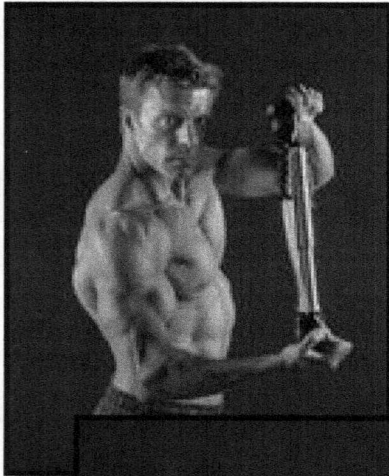

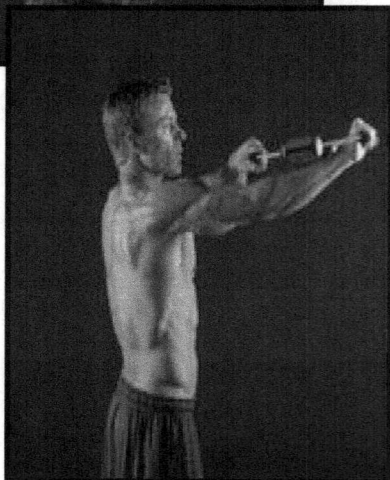

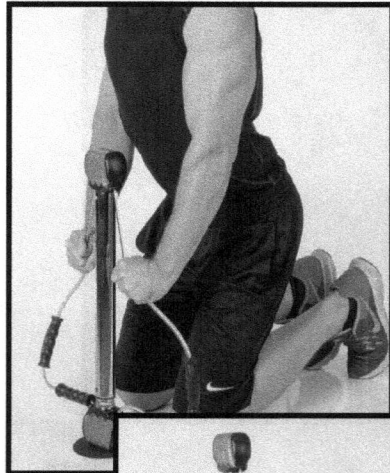

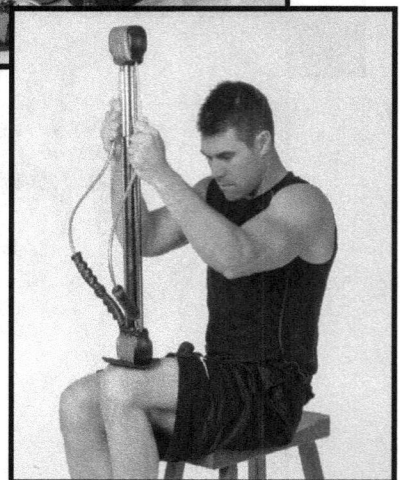

CHAPTER 9
REP RANGE X4
MUSCLE-SURGE PROGRAM
PHASE 1
WEEK 1 OF 3

REP SPEED CONTRACT 2 SECONDS, RELEASE 2 SECONDS
PERFORM EACH PHASE FOR ONE WEEK EACH

MUSCLE-SURGE

09 REP RANGE MUSCLE-SURGE PROGRAM

REP RANGE MUSCLE-SURGE PROGRAM " MUSCLE-BUILDING PHASE"

WEEK 1: 20x15 Perform 20 reps followed by a 15 second isometric contraction, 2-3 rounds.

WEEK 2: 30x30 Perform 30 reps followed by a 30 second isometric contraction. 2 sets per exercise.

WEEK 3: 15x30 Perform 15 reps followed by a 30 second isometric contraction. 2 set per exercise

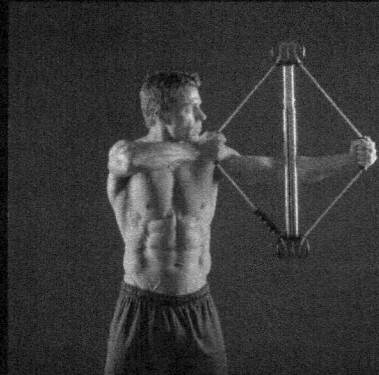

MUSCLE-SURGE

09 REP RANGE MUSCLE-SURGE PROGRAM

HOW TO PERFORM THIS ROUTINE:
PHASE ONE 20x15 PHASE

Perform 20 reps followed by a 15 second isometric contraction 2-3 rounds.

DAY ONE

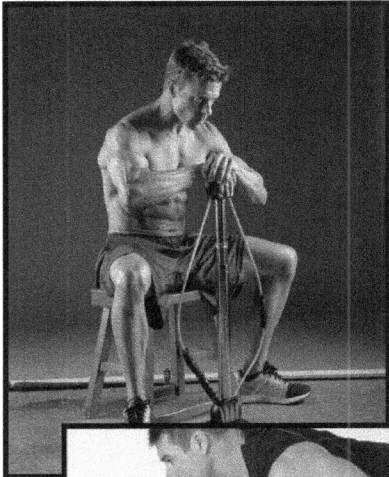

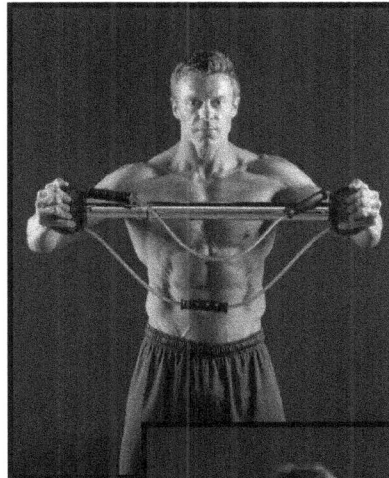

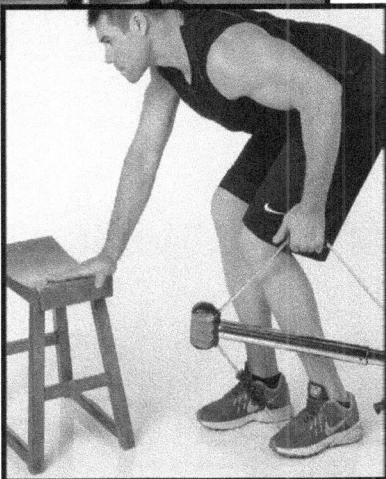

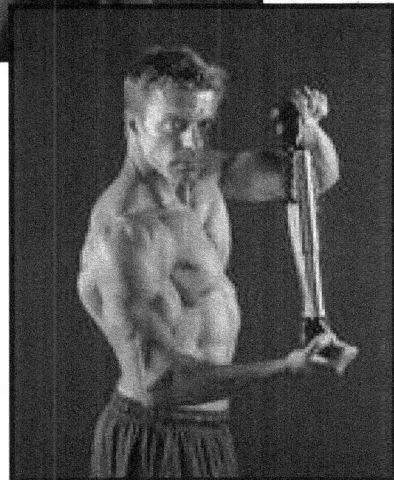

MUSCLE-SURGE

09 REP RANGE MUSCLE-SURGE PROGRAM

HOW TO PERFORM THIS ROUTINE:
PHASE ONE 20x15 PHASE

Perform 20 reps followed by a 15 second isometric contraction 2-3 rounds.

DAY ONE continued............

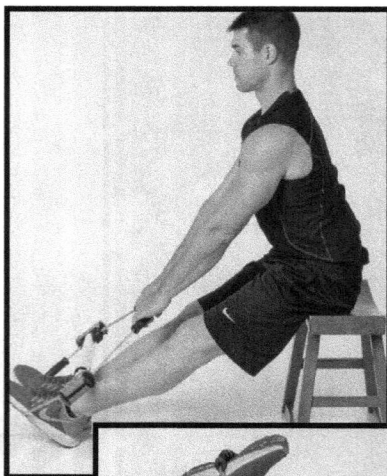

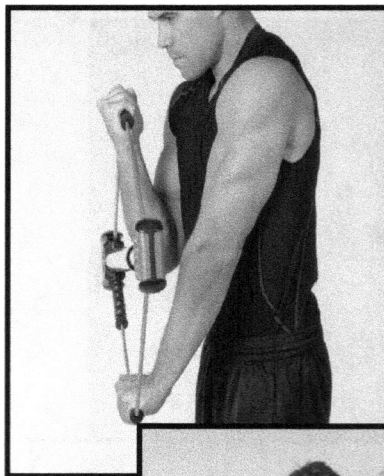

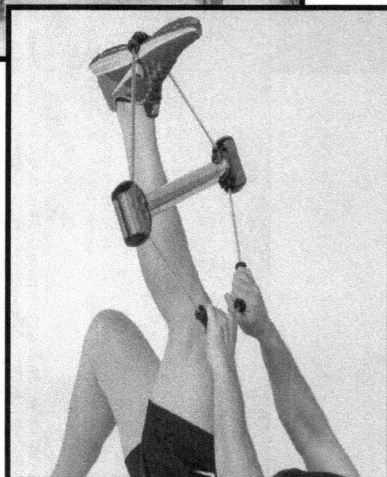

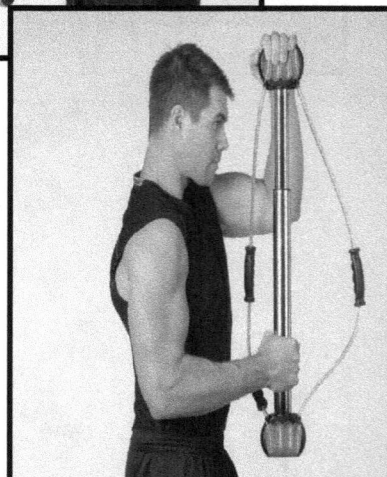

MUSCLE-SURGE

09 REP RANGE MUSCLE-SURGE PROGRAM

HOW TO PERFORM THIS ROUTINE:
PHASE ONE 20x15 PHASE

Perform 20 reps followed by a 15 second isometric contraction 2-3 rounds.

DAY TWO

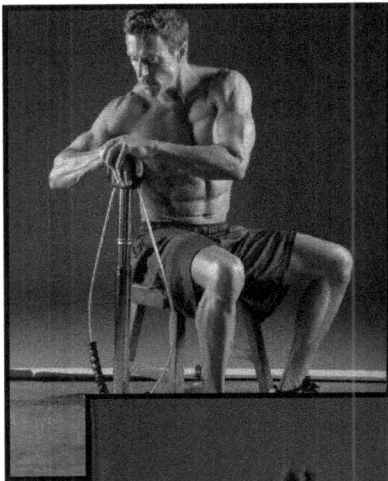

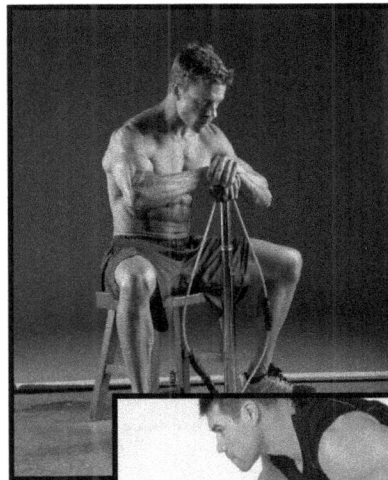

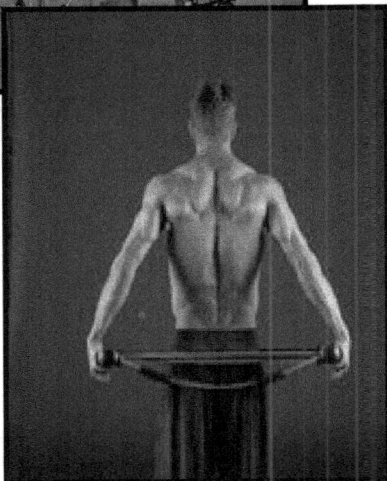

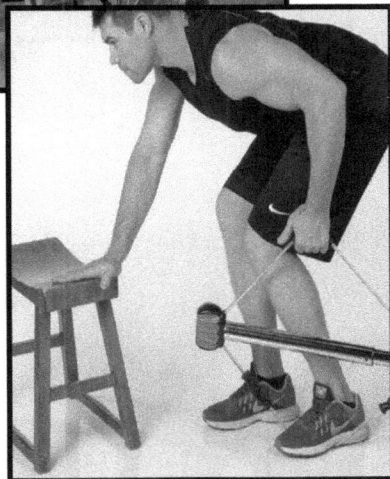

MUSCLE-SURGE

09 REP RANGE MUSCLE-SURGE PROGRAM

HOW TO PERFORM THIS ROUTINE:
PHASE ONE 20x15 PHASE

Perform 20 reps followed by a 15 second isometric contraction 2-3 rounds.

DAY TWO continued.......

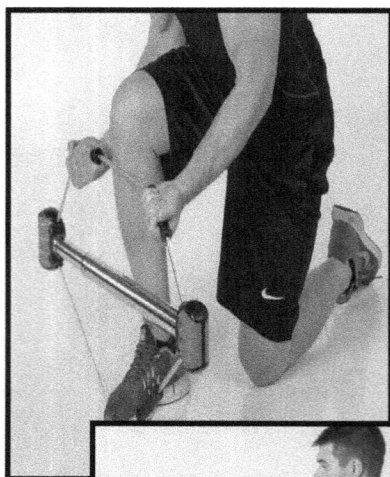

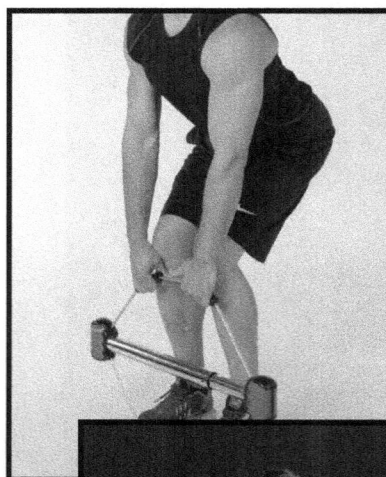

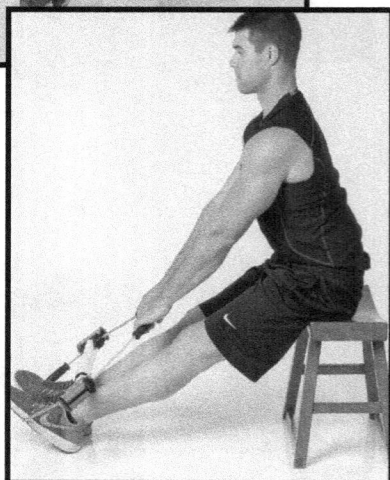

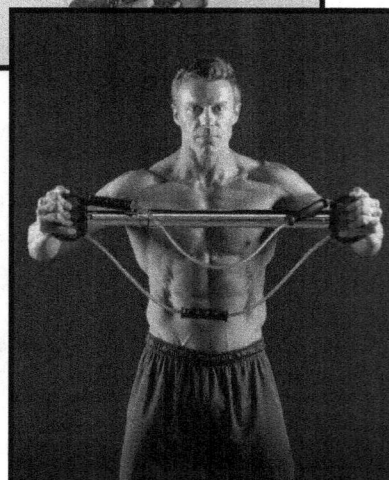

MUSCLE-SURGE

09 REP RANGE MUSCLE-SURGE PROGRAM

HOW TO PERFORM THIS ROUTINE:
PHASE ONE 20x15 PHASE

Perform 20 reps followed by a 15 second isometric contraction 2-3 rounds.

DAY THREE

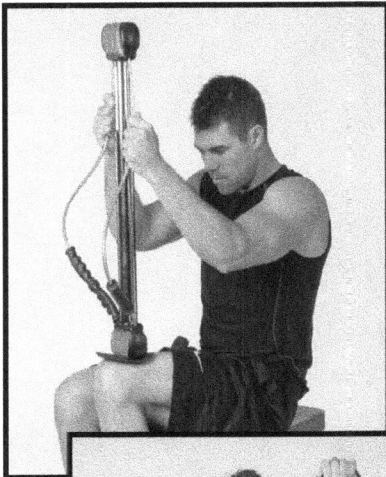

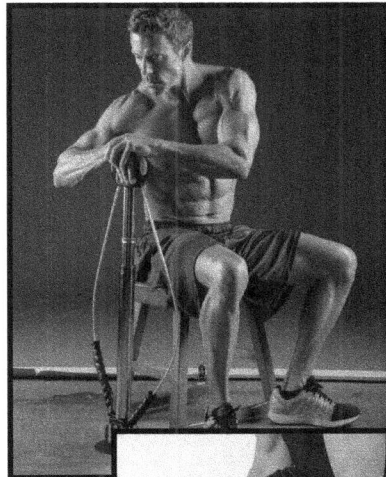

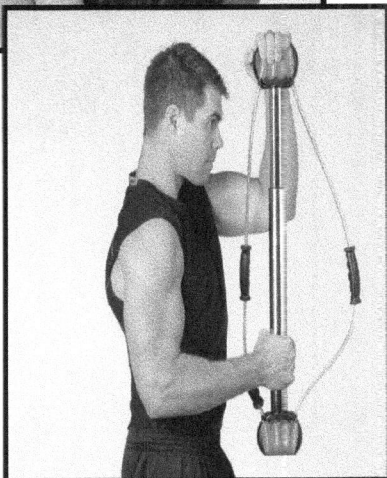

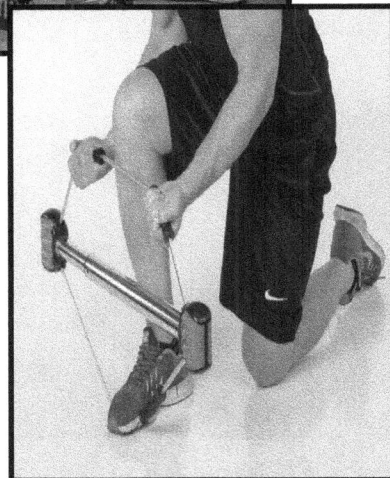

MUSCLE-SURGE

09 REP RANGE MUSCLE-SURGE PROGRAM

HOW TO PERFORM THIS ROUTINE:
PHASE ONE 20x15 PHASE
Perform 20 reps followed by a 15 second isometric contraction 2-3 rounds.

DAY THREE continued..........

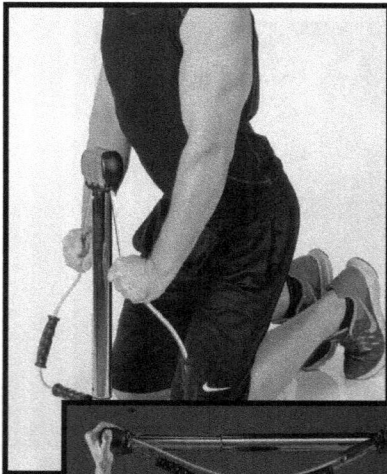

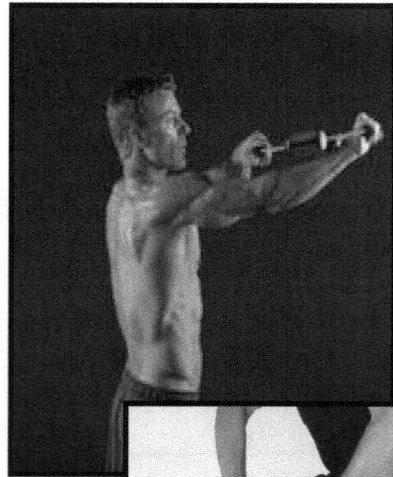

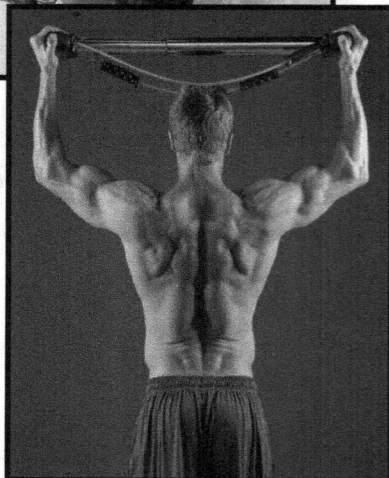

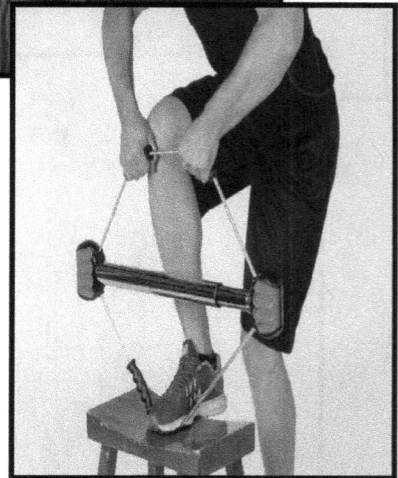

MUSCLE-SURGE

09 REP RANGE MUSCLE-SURGE PROGRAM

HOW TO PERFORM THIS ROUTINE:
PHASE ONE 20x15 PHASE

Perform 20 reps followed by a 15 second isometric contraction 2-3 rounds.

DAY FOUR

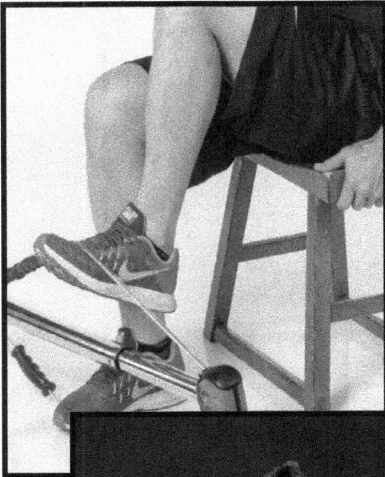

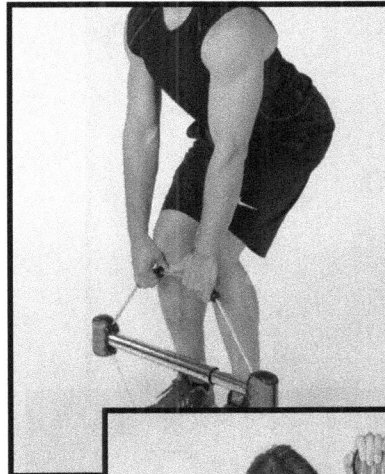

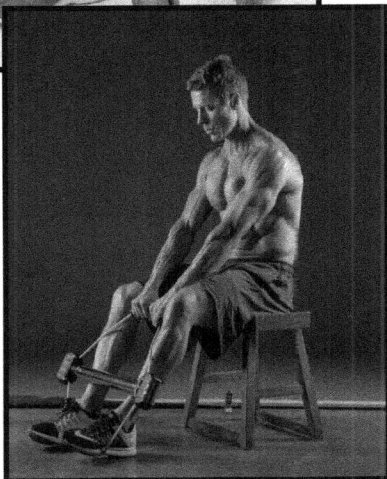

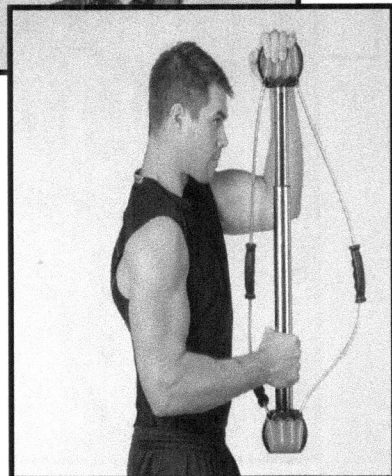

MUSCLE-SURGE

09 REP RANGE MUSCLE-SURGE PROGRAM

HOW TO PERFORM THIS ROUTINE:
PHASE ONE 20x15 PHASE
Perform 20 reps followed by a 15 second isometric contraction 2-3 rounds.

DAY FOUR continued...........

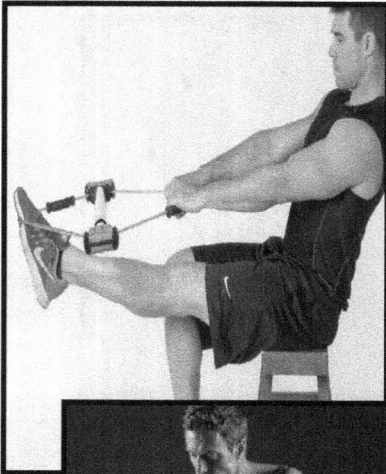

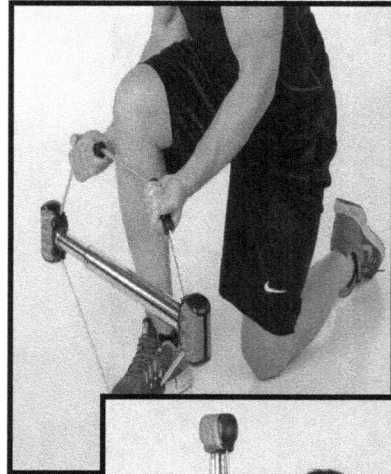

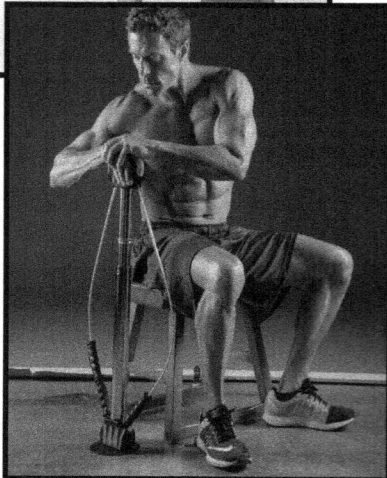

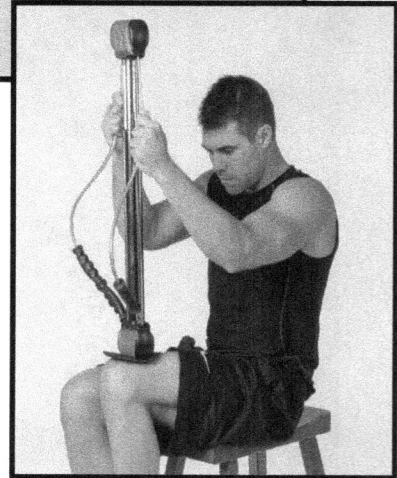

MUSCLE-SURGE

09 REP RANGE MUSCLE-SURGE PROGRAM

HOW TO PERFORM THIS ROUTINE:
PHASE ONE 20x15 PHASE

Perform 20 reps followed by a 15 second isometric contraction 2-3 rounds.

DAY FIVE

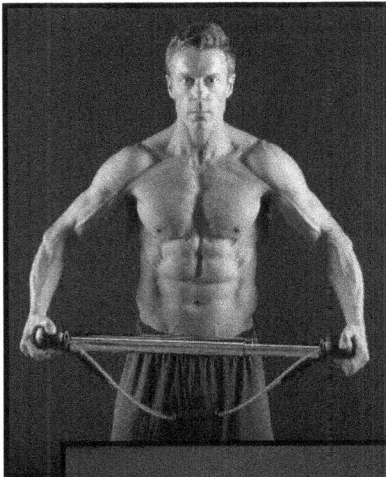
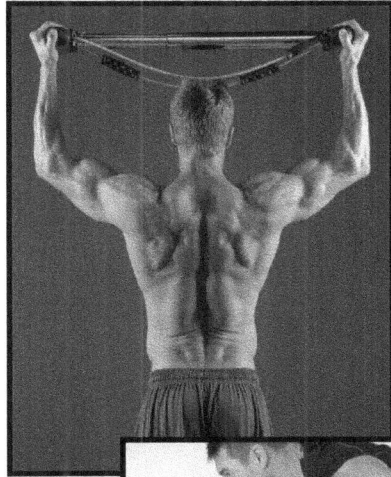
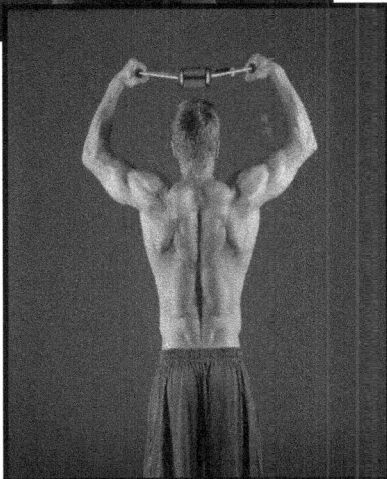
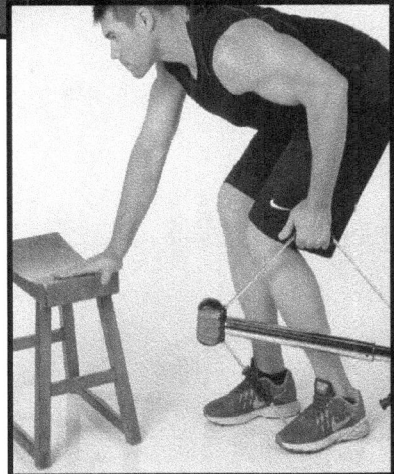

MUSCLE-SURGE

09 REP RANGE MUSCLE-SURGE PROGRAM

HOW TO PERFORM THIS ROUTINE:
PHASE ONE 20x15 PHASE

Perform 20 reps followed by a 15 second isometric contraction 2-3 rounds.

DAY FIVE continued.............

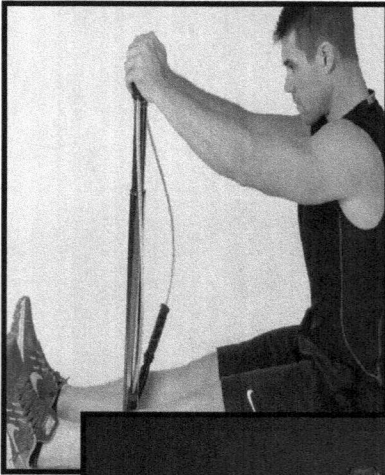

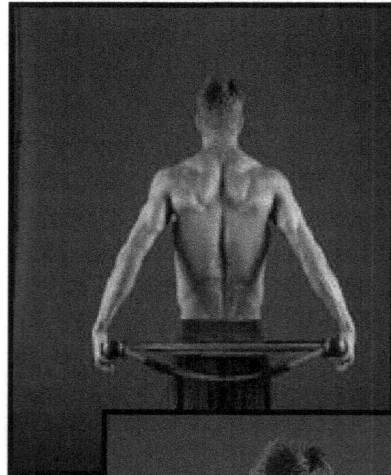

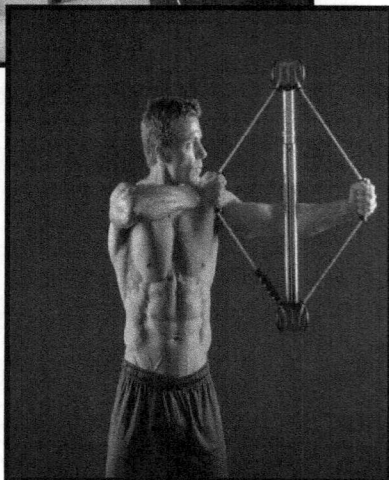

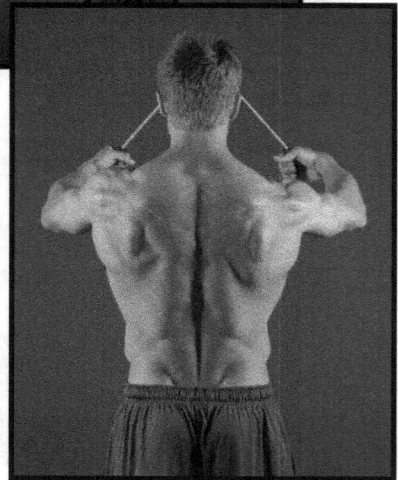

CHAPTER 9

REP RANGE

MUSCLE SURGE X4

PHASE 2

WEEK 2 OF 3

REP SPEED CONTRACT 2 SECONDS, RELEASE 2 SECONDS

MUSCLE-SURGE

09 REP RANGE MUSCLE-SURGE PROGRAM

HOW TO PERFORM THIS ROUTINE:
PHASE TWO 30X30 PHASE

Perform 30 reps followed by a 30 second isometric contraction, 2 rounds.

DAY ONE

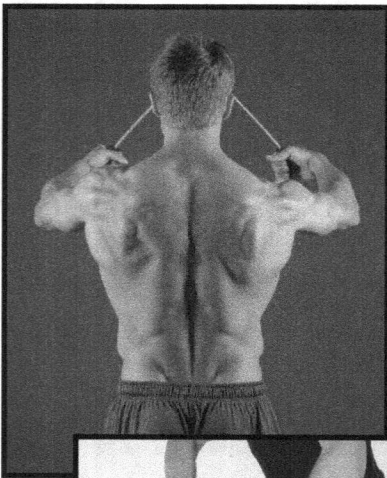
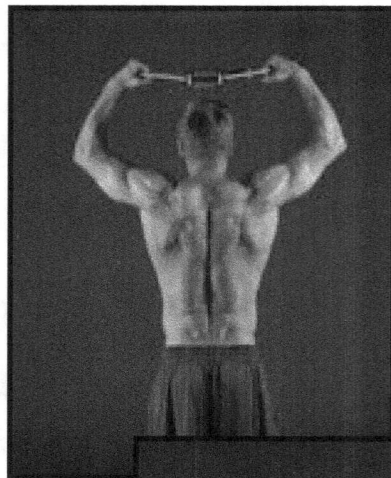
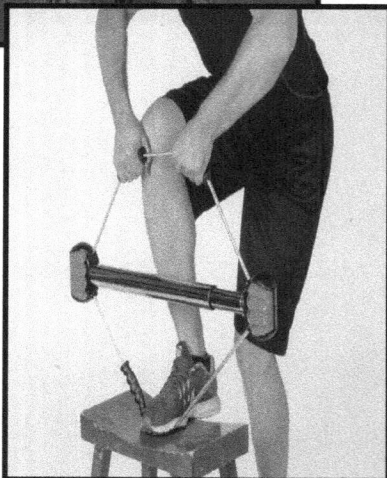
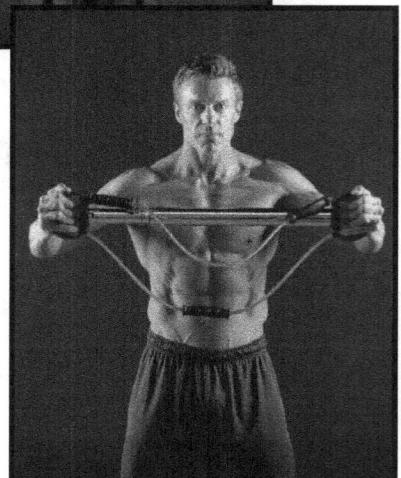

MUSCLE-SURGE

09 REP RANGE MUSCLE-SURGE PROGRAM

HOW TO PERFORM THIS ROUTINE:
PHASE TWO 30X30 PHASE
Perform 30 reps followed by a 30 second isometric contraction, 2 rounds.

DAY ONE continued..........

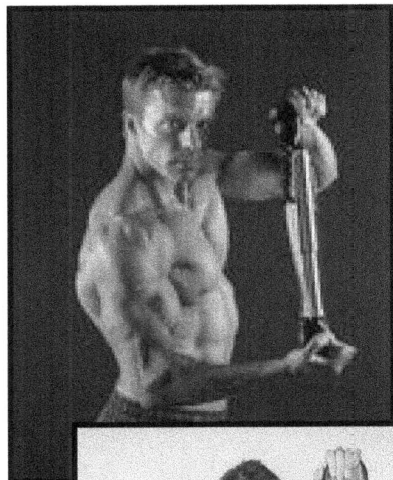

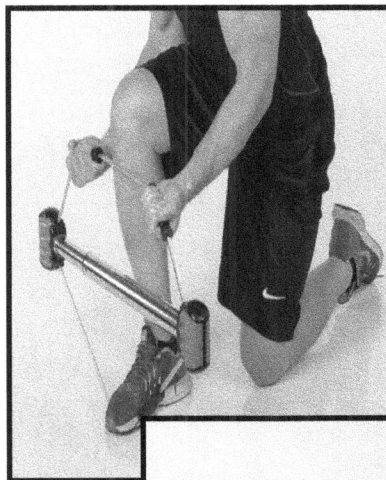

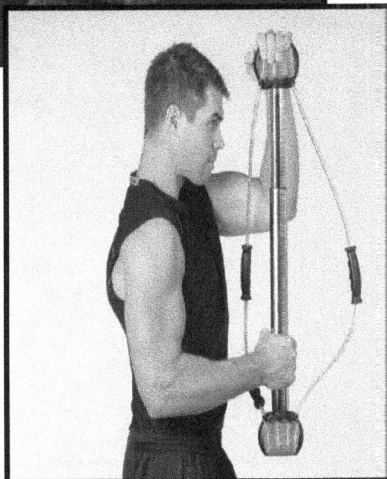

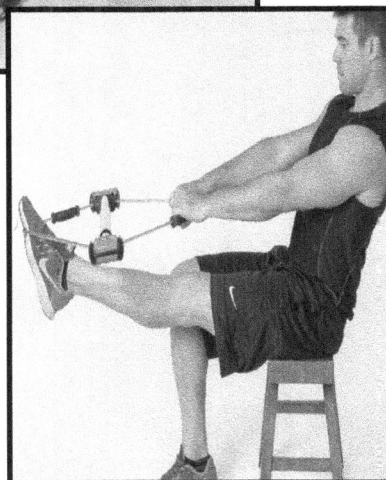

MUSCLE-SURGE

09 REP RANGE MUSCLE-SURGE PROGRAM

HOW TO PERFORM THIS ROUTINE:
PHASE TWO 30X30 PHASE
Perform 30 reps followed by a 30 second isometric contraction, 2 rounds.

DAY TWO

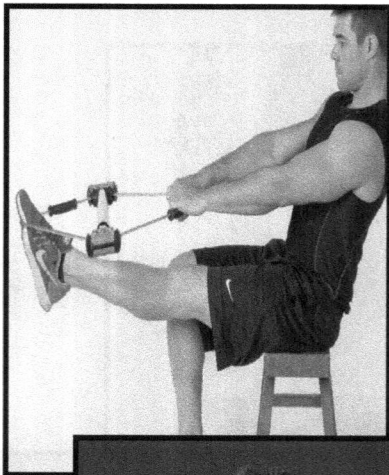
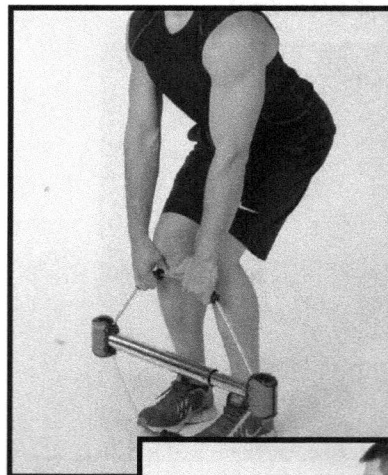
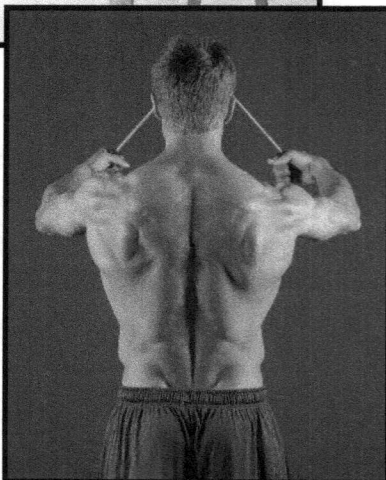
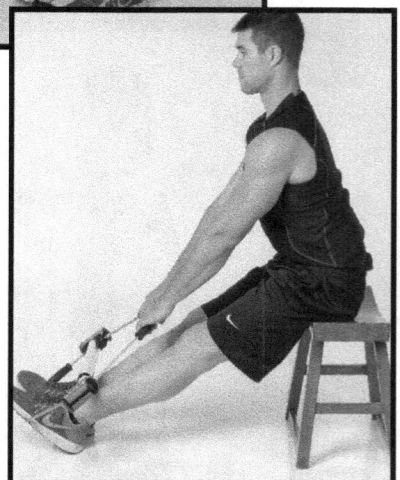

MUSCLE-SURGE

09 REP RANGE MUSCLE-SURGE PROGRAM

HOW TO PERFORM THIS ROUTINE:
PHASE TWO 30X30 PHASE

Perform 30 reps followed by a 30 second isometric contraction...2 rounds.

DAY TWO contin.......

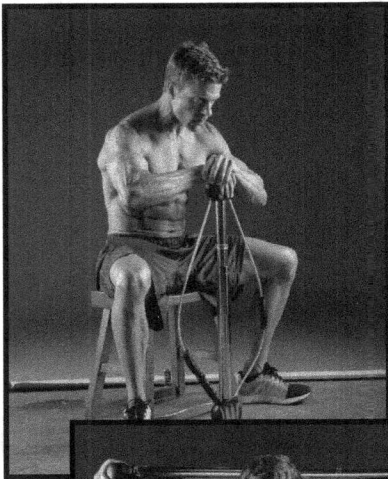

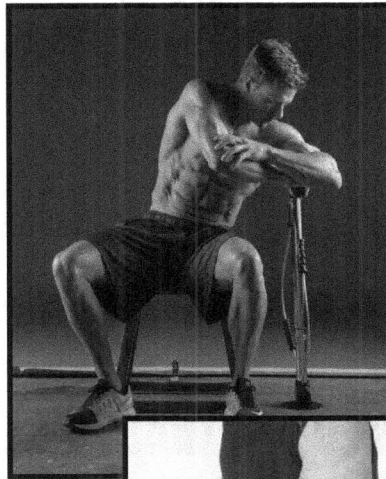

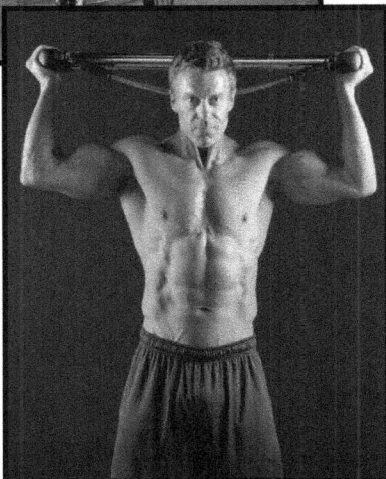

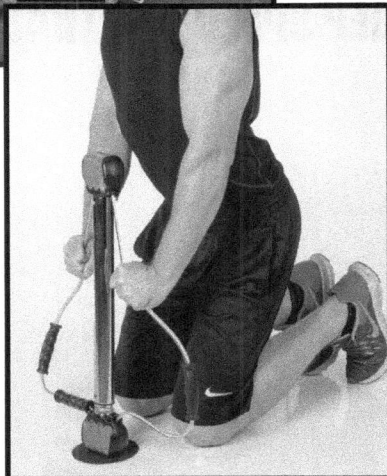

CHAPTER 9
REP RANGE
MUSCLE-SURGE X4
PHASE 3
WEEK 3 OF 3
REP SPEED CONTRACT 2 SECONDS, RELEASE 2 SECONDS

MUSCLE-SURGE

09 REP RANGE MUSCLE-SURGE PROGRAM

HOW TO PERFORM THIS ROUTINE:
PHASE THREE 15x30 PHASE

Perform 15 reps followed by a 30 second isometric contraction....2 rounds.

DAY ONE

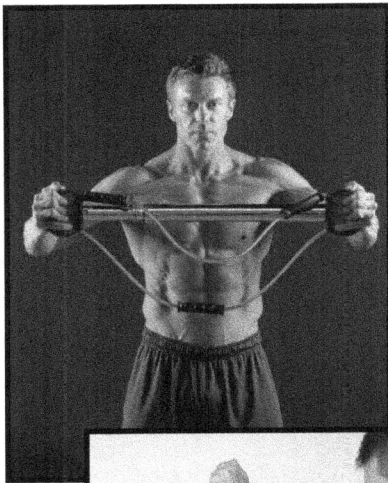

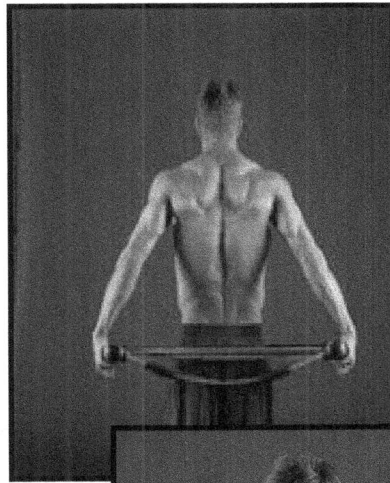

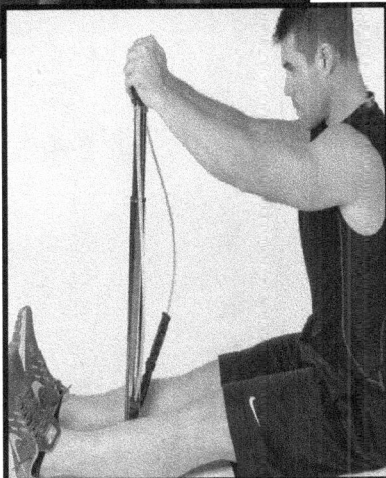

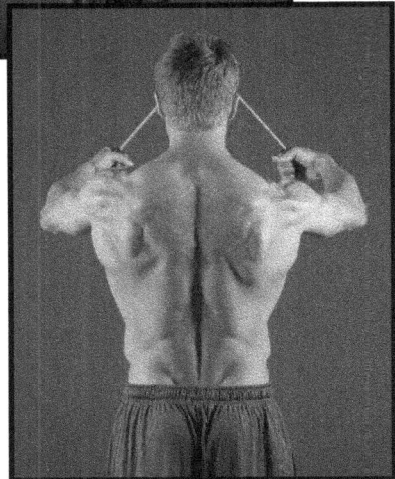

MUSCLE-SURGE

09 REP RANGE MUSCLE-SURGE PROGRAM

HOW TO PERFORM THIS ROUTINE:
PHASE THREE 15x30 PHASE
Perform 15 reps followed by a 30 second isometric contraction...2 rounds.

DAY ONE continued............

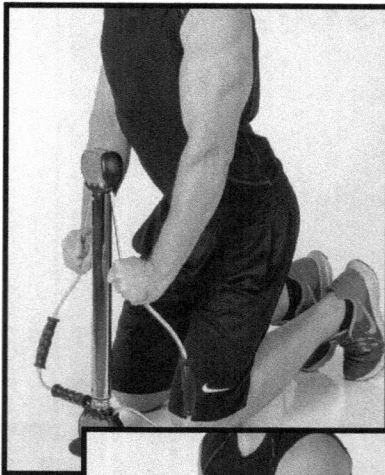

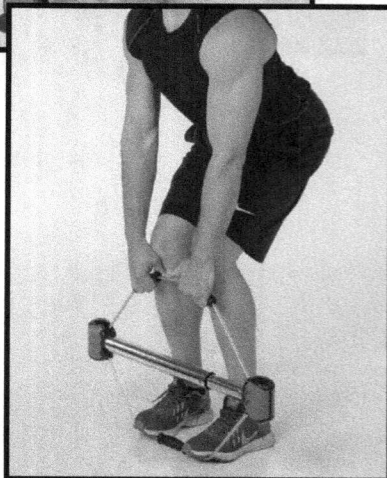

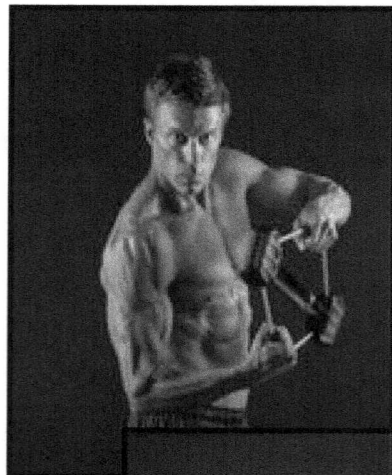

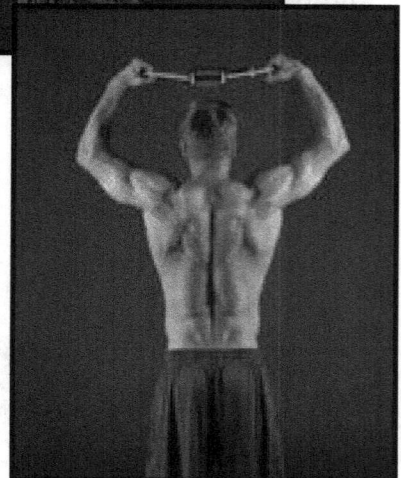

MUSCLE-SURGE

09 REP RANGE MUSCLE-SURGE PROGRAM

HOW TO PERFORM THIS ROUTINE:
PHASE THREE 15x30 PHASE
Perform 15 reps followed by a 30 second isometric contraction...2 rounds.

DAY TWO

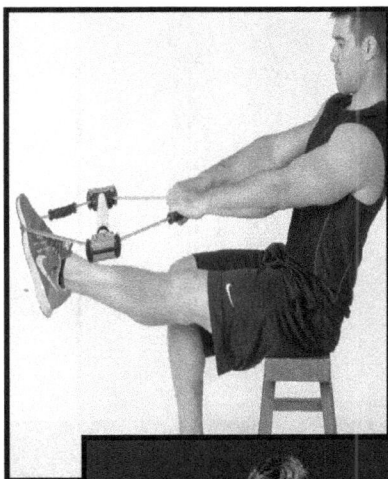

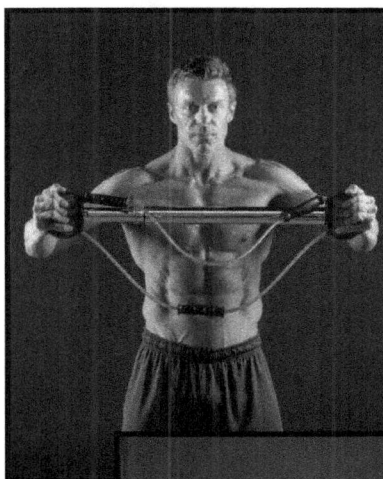

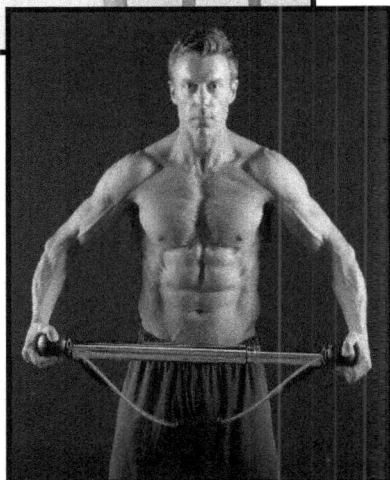

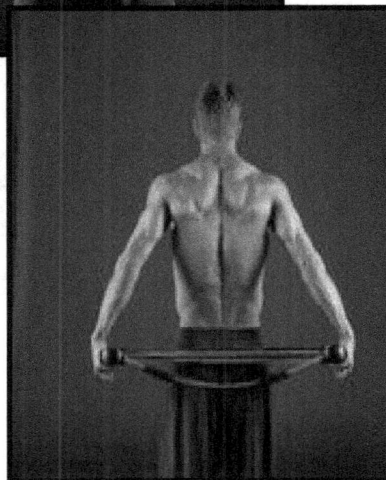

MUSCLE-SURGE

09 REP RANGE MUSCLE-SURGE PROGRAM

HOW TO PERFORM THIS ROUTINE:
PHASE THREE 15x30 PHASE

Perform 15 reps followed by a 30 second isometric contraction...2 rounds.

DAY TWO continued..........

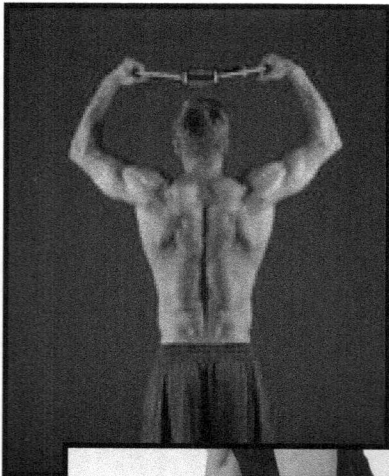

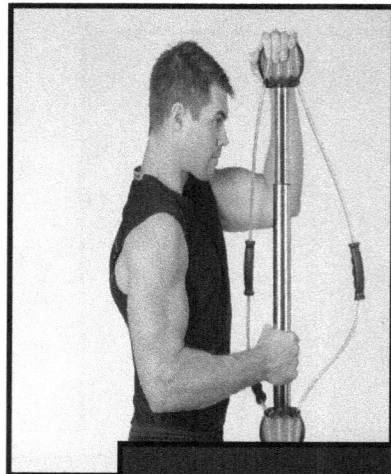

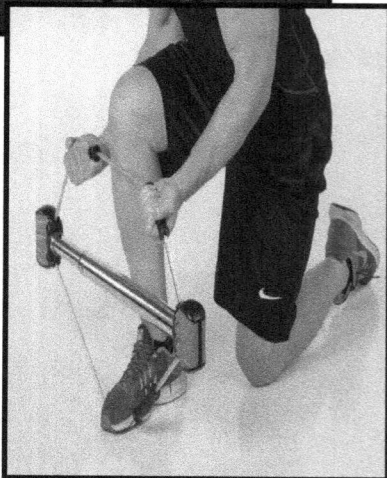

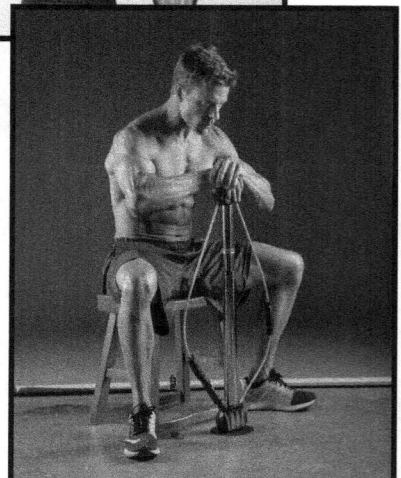

CHAPTER 10
MUSCLE-SURGE
POWER 7 X4
PHASE 13

PERFORM 7 REPS, EACH REP IS HELD FOR 1 SECOND 4 WEEKS

MUSCLE-SURGE

10 POWER 7 PROGRAM

HOW TO PERFORM THIS ROUTINE:
THE POWER 7 PROGRAM

Perform the **POWER 7 WORKOUT**—by performing 7 reps. Each rep is held for 1 second. Perform all exercises one after the other until all exercises are completed without rest. Perform 2 rounds of these between each round rest for 5 seconds before starting another round.
Alternate day one and day two for 6 days per week.

DAY ONE

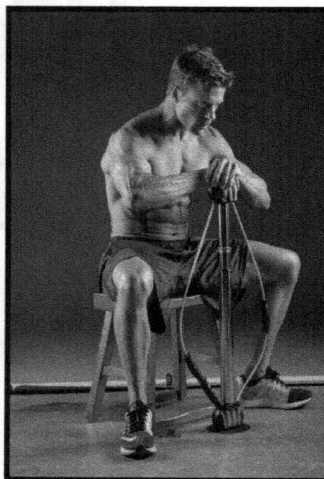
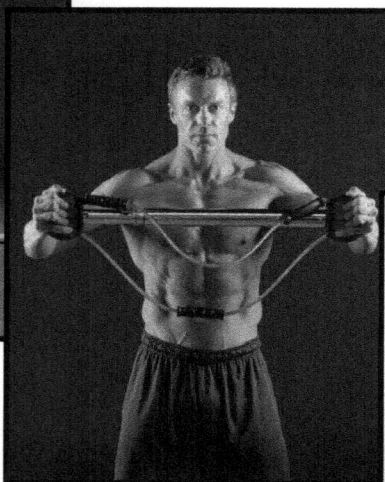
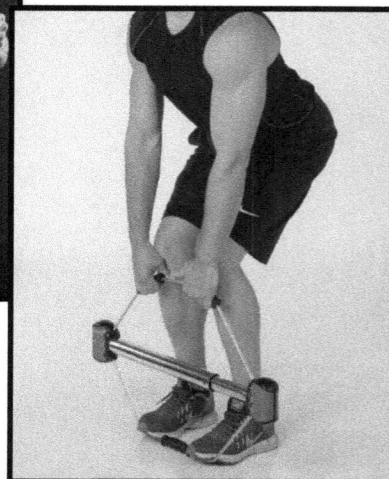

MUSCLE-SURGE

10 POWER 7 PROGRAM

HOW TO PERFORM THIS ROUTINE:
THE POWER 7 PROGRAM

Perform the **POWER 7 WORKOUT**—by performing 7 reps. Each rep is held for 1 second. Perform all exercises one after the other until all exercises are completed without rest. Perform 2 rounds of these between each round rest for 5 seconds before starting another round.
Alternate day one and day two for 6 days per week.

DAY ONE continued..........

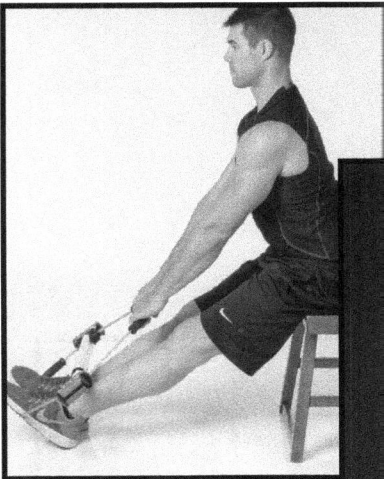

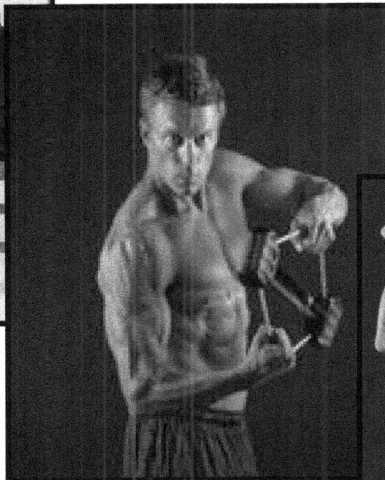

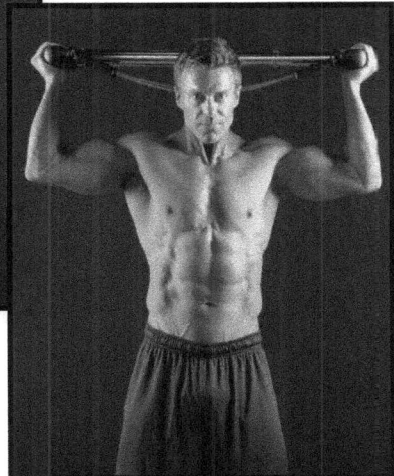

MUSCLE-SURGE

10 POWER 7 PROGRAM

HOW TO PERFORM THIS ROUTINE:
THE POWER 7 PROGRAM

Perform the **POWER 7 WORKOUT**—by performing 7 reps. Each rep is held for 1second. Perform all exercises one after the other until all exercises are completed without rest. Perform 2 rounds of these between each round rest for 5 seconds before starting another round.
Alternate day one and day two for 6 days per week.

DAY ONE continued......

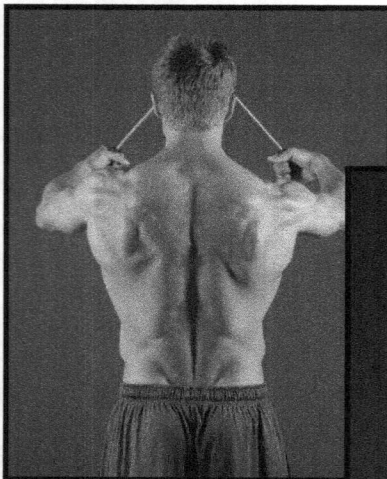

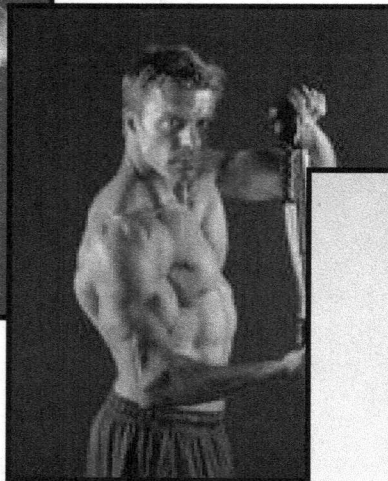

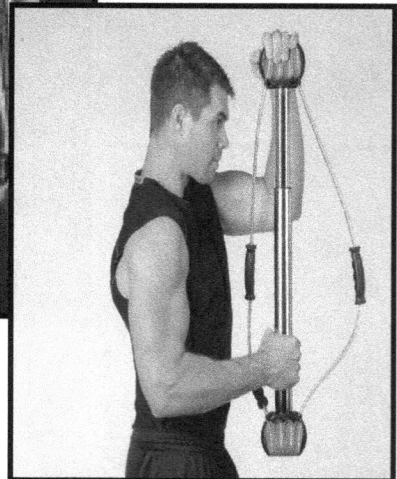

MUSCLE-SURGE

10 POWER 7 PROGRAM

HOW TO PERFORM THIS ROUTINE:
THE POWER 7 PROGRAM

Perform the **POWER 7 WORKOUT**—by performing 7 reps. Each rep is held for 1 second. Perform all exercises one after the other until all exercises are completed without rest. Perform 2 rounds of these between each round rest for 5 seconds before starting another round.
Alternate day one and day two for 6 days per week.

DAY TWO

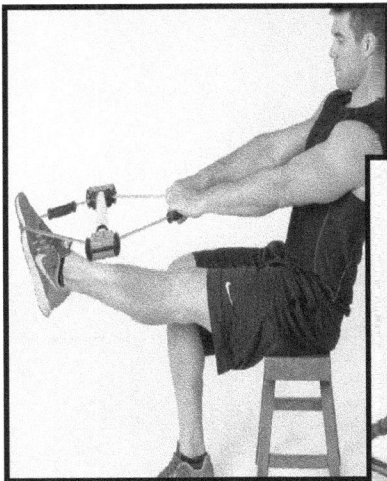
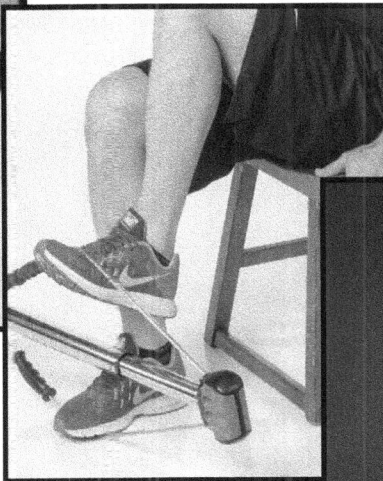
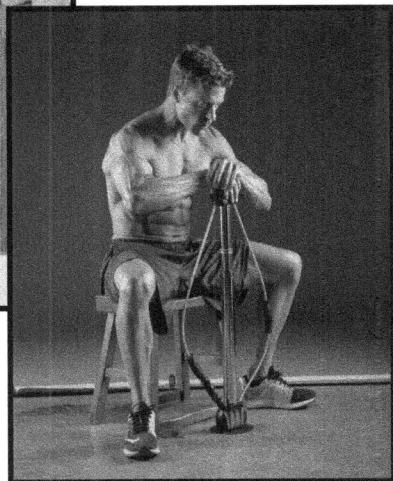

MUSCLE-SURGE

10 POWER 7 PROGRAM

HOW TO PERFORM THIS ROUTINE:
THE POWER 7 PROGRAM

Perform the **POWER 7 WORKOUT**—by performing 7 reps. Each rep is held for 1second. Perform all exercises one after the other until all exercises are completed without rest. Perform 2 rounds of these between each round rest for 5 seconds before starting another round.
Alternate day one and day two for 6 days per week.

DAY TWO continue........

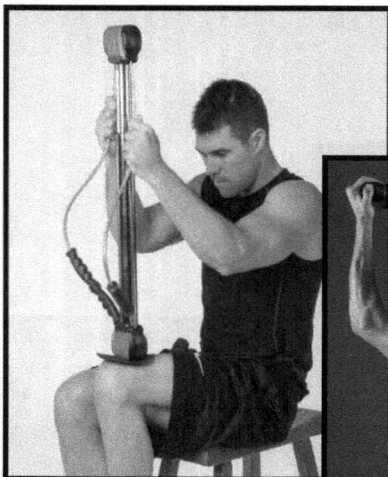

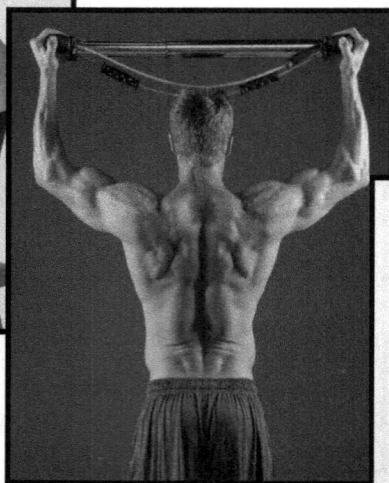

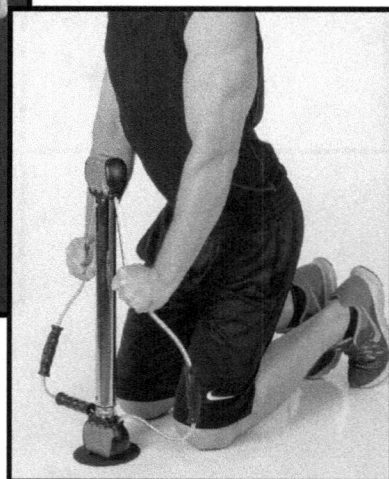

MUSCLE-SURGE

10 POWER 7 PROGRAM

HOW TO PERFORM THIS ROUTINE:
THE POWER 7 PROGRAM

Perform the **POWER 7 WORKOUT**—by performing 7 reps. Each rep is held for 1second. Perform all exercises one after the other until all exercises are completed without rest. Perform 2 rounds of these between each round rest for 5 seconds before starting another round.
Alternate day one and day two for 6 days per week.

DAY TWO continued...........

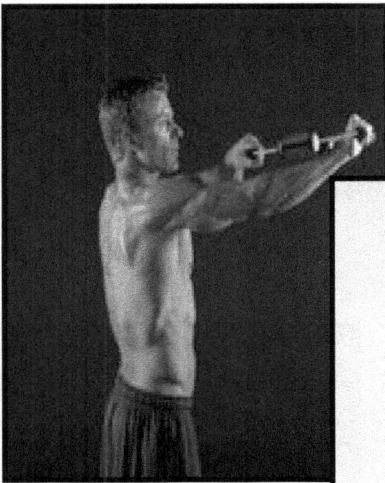

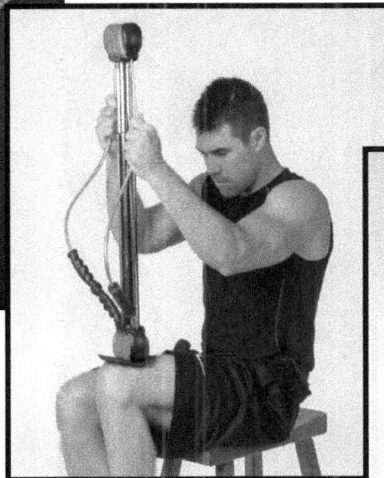

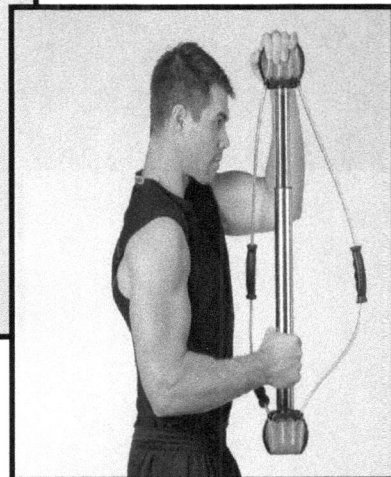

MUSCLE-SURGE

10 POWER 7 PROGRAM

HOW TO PERFORM THIS ROUTINE:
THE POWER 7 PROGRAM

Perform the **POWER 7 WORKOUT**—by performing 7 reps. Each rep is held for 1second. Perform all exercises one after the other until all exercises are completed without rest. Perform 2 rounds of these between each round rest for 5 seconds before starting another round.
Alternate day one and day two for 6 days per week.

DAY TWO continued..........

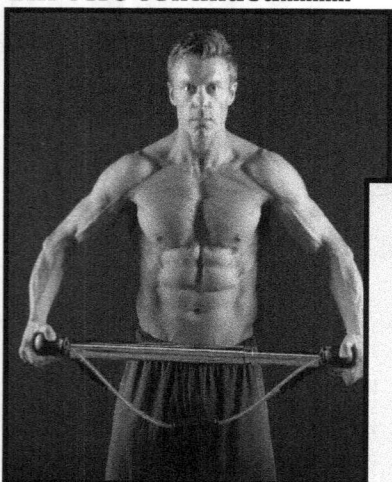

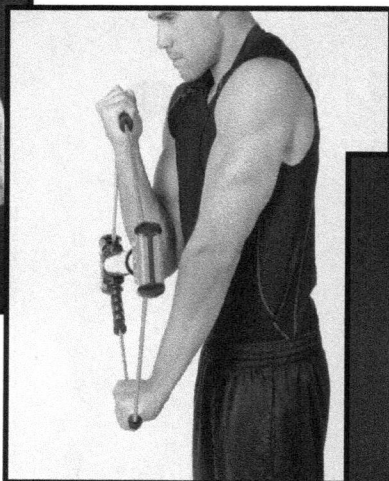

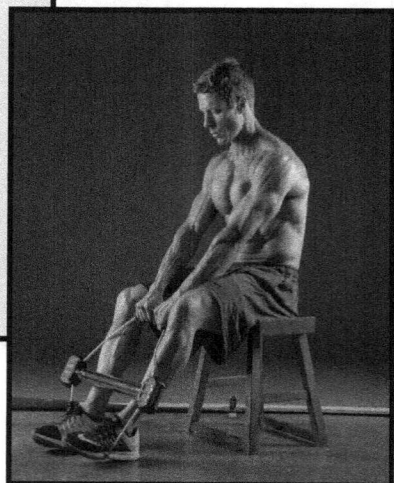

CHAPTER 11
POWER REP RANGE X2
MUSCLE-SURGE
PHASE ONE

REP RANGES CHANGE THROUGHOUT THE WEEK

POWER REP RANGE X2

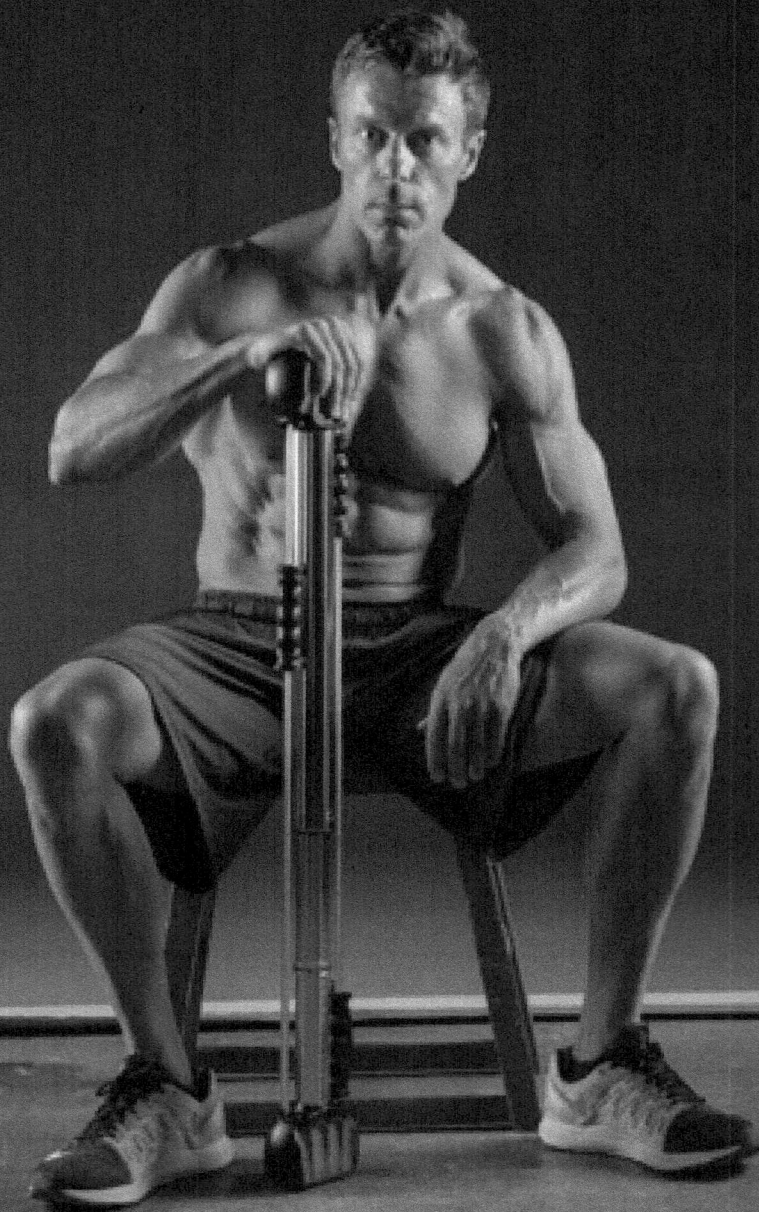

POWER REP RANGE X2

11 POWER REP RANGE X2 PHASE ONE

HOW TO PERFORM THIS ROUTINE:
POWER REP RANGE X2

Day 1=10 reps, Day 2=30 reps, Day 3=15 reps, Day 4=7 reps, Day 5=20 reps
Day 6=10 reps, Day 7=30 reps. On the last rep perform a 5 second
Isometric contraction. Perform all exercises without rest for 3 rounds.
Perform this routine every day 7 days per week for 4 weeks

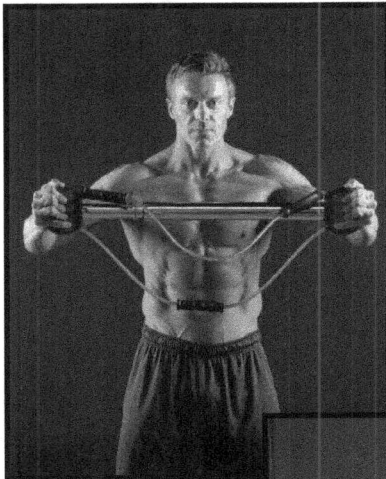

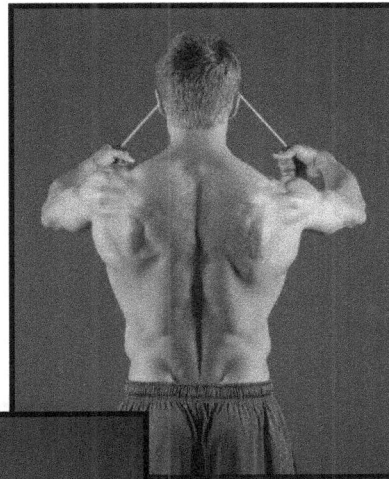

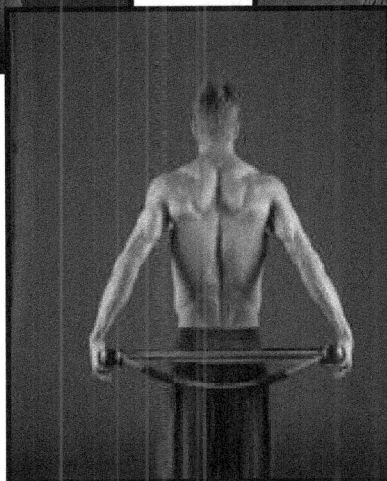

POWER REP RANGE X2

11 POWER REP RANGE X2 PHASE ONE

HOW TO PERFORM THIS ROUTINE:
POWER REP RANGE X2

Day 1=10 reps, Day 2=30 reps, Day 3=15 reps, Day 4=7 reps, Day 5=20 reps
Day 6=10 reps, Day 7=30 reps. On the last rep perform a 5 second
Isometric contraction. Perform all exercises without rest for 3 rounds.
Perform this routine every day 7 days per week for 4 weeks

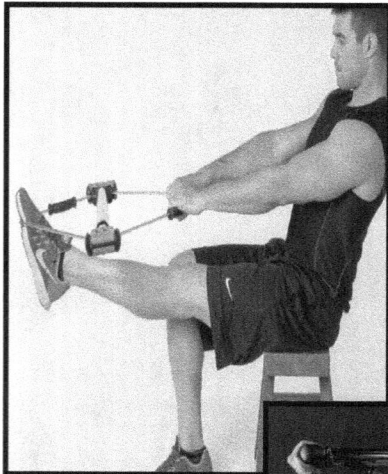

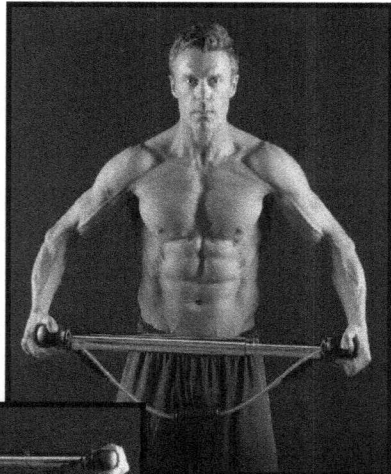

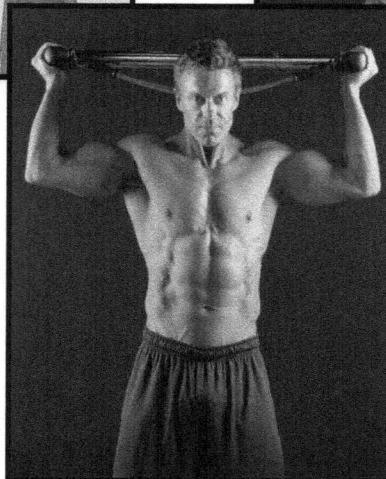

POWER REP RANGE X2

11 POWER REP RANGE X2 PHASE ONE

HOW TO PERFORM THIS ROUTINE:
POWER REP RANGE X2

Day 1=10 reps, Day 2=30 reps, Day 3=15 reps, Day 4=7 reps, Day 5=20 reps
Day 6=10 reps, Day 7=30 reps. On the last rep perform a 5 second
Isometric contraction. Perform all exercises without rest for 3 rounds.
Perform this routine every day 7 days per week for 4 weeks

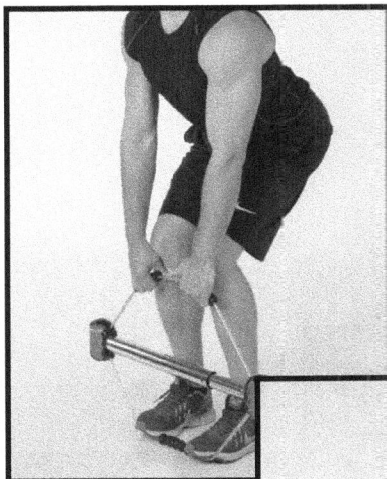

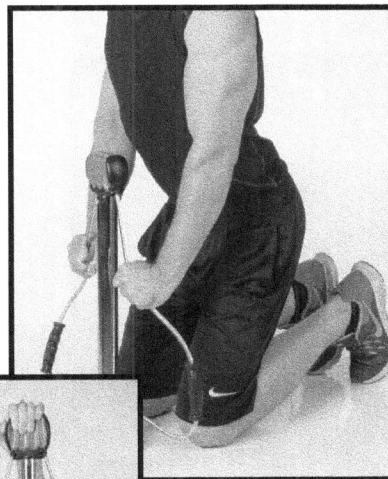

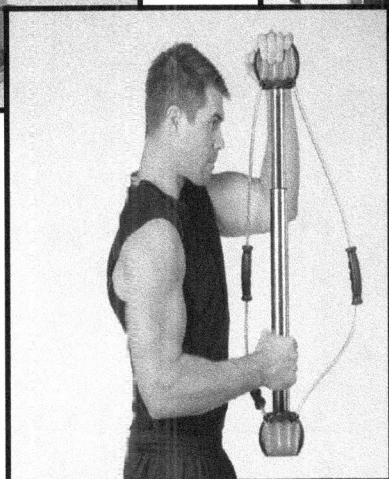

PHASE TWO

11 POWER REP RANGE X2 PHASE TWO

HOW TO PERFORM THIS ROUTINE:
POWER REP RANGE X2

Day 1=7-9 reps, Day 2=20 reps, Day 3=30 reps, Day 4=30 reps, Day 5=9 reps
Day 6=15 reps, Day 7=30 reps. On the last rep perform a 10 second
Isometric contraction. Perform all exercises without rest for 2 rounds.
Alternate day 1 and day 2.....7 days per week for 4 weeks

DAY ONE

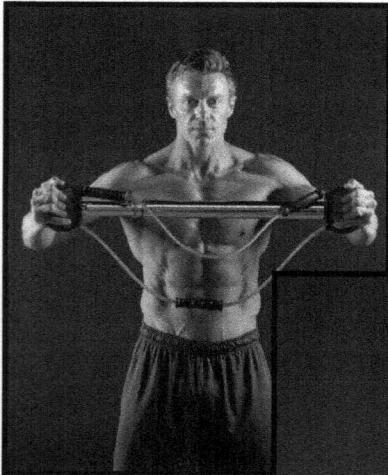
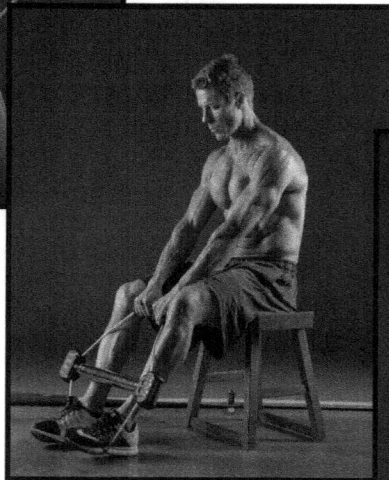
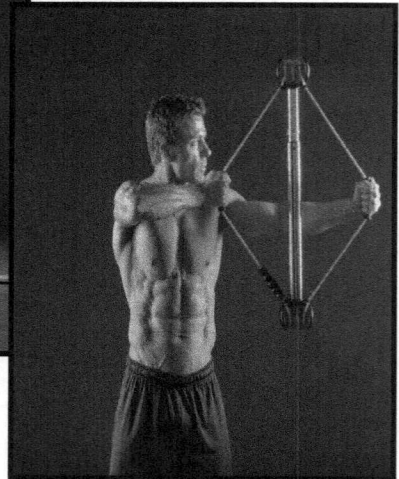

PHASE TWO

11 POWER REP RANGE X2 PHASE TWO

HOW TO PERFORM THIS ROUTINE:
POWER REP RANGE X2

Day 1=7-9 reps, Day 2=20 reps, Day 3=30 reps, Day 4=30 reps, Day 5=9 reps
Day 6=15 reps, Day 7=30 reps. On the last rep perform a 10 second
Isometric contraction. Perform all exercises without rest for 2 rounds.
Alternate day 1 and day 2.... 7 days per week for 4 weeks

DAY ONE continued.........

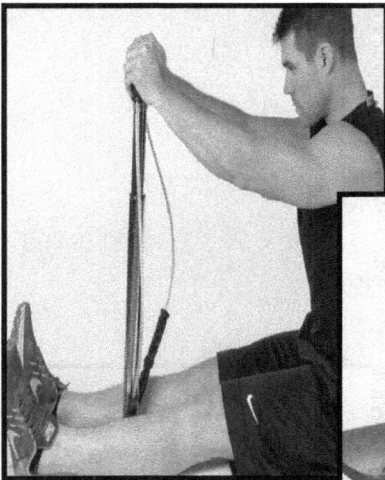

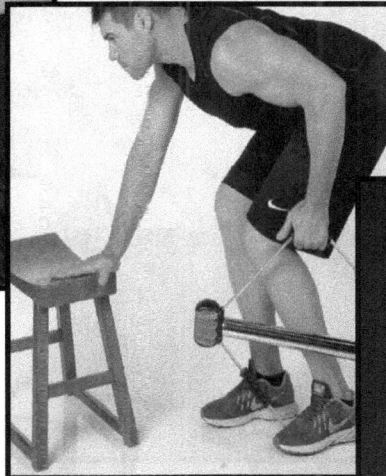

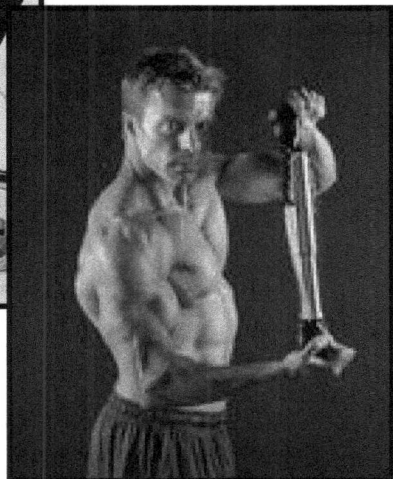

PHASE TWO

11 POWER REP RANGE X2 PHASE TWO

HOW TO PERFORM THIS ROUTINE:
POWER REP RANGE X2

Day 1=7-9 reps, Day 2=20 reps, Day 3=30 reps, Day 4=30 reps, Day 5=9 reps
Day 6=15 reps, Day 7=30 reps. On the last rep perform a 10 second
Isometric contraction. Perform all exercises without rest for 2 rounds.
Alternate day 1 and day 2......7 days per week for 4 weeks

DAY ONE contin........

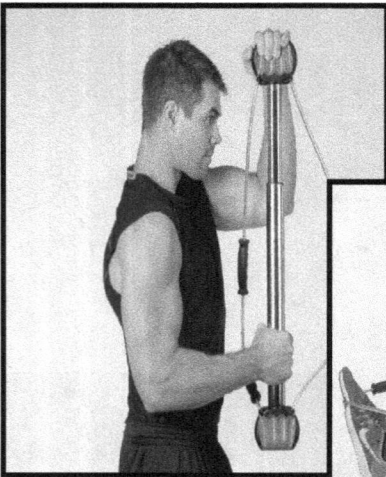

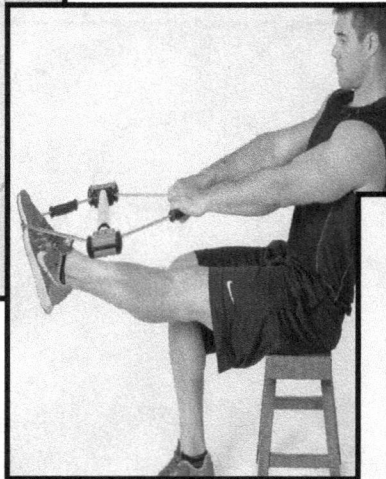

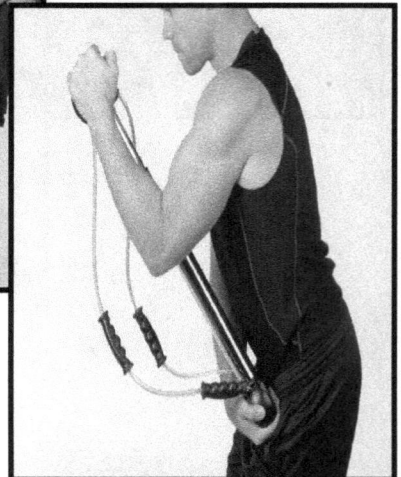

PHASE TWO

11 ISO-POWER REP RANGE X2 PHASE TWO

HOW TO PERFORM THIS ROUTINE:
POWER REP RANGE X2

Day 1=7-9 reps, Day 2=20 reps, Day 3=30 reps, Day 4=30 reps, Day 5=9 reps
Day 6=15 reps, Day 7=30 reps. On the last rep perform a 10 second
Isometric contraction. Perform all exercises without rest for 2 rounds.
Alternate day 1 and day 2......7 days per week for 4 weeks

DAY TWO

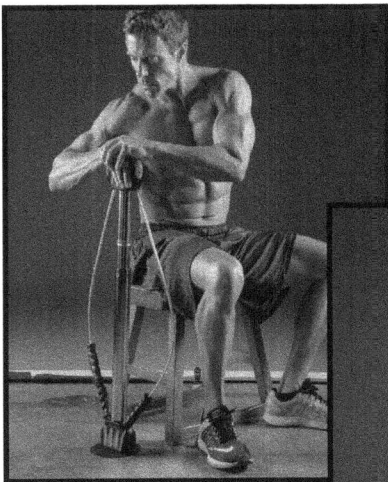
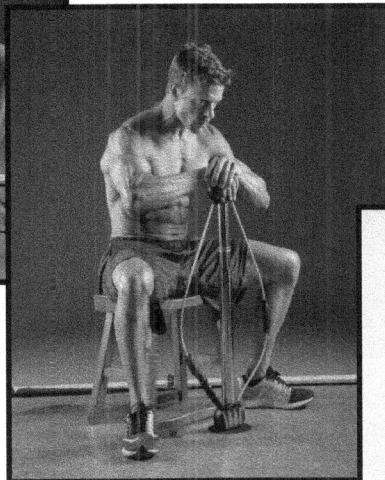
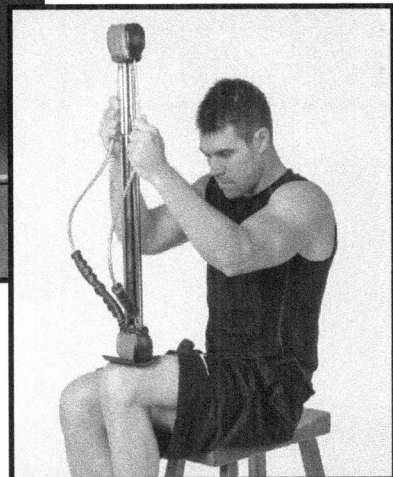

PHASE TWO

11 POWER REP RANGE X2 PHASE TWO

HOW TO PERFORM THIS ROUTINE:
POWER REP RANGE X2

Day 1=7-9 reps, Day 2=20 reps, Day 3=30 reps, Day 4=30 reps, Day 5=9 reps
Day 6=15 reps, Day 7=30 reps. On the last rep perform a 10 second
Isometric contraction. Perform all exercises without rest for 2 rounds.
Alternate day 1 and day 2......7 days per week for 4 weeks

DAY TWO continued...........

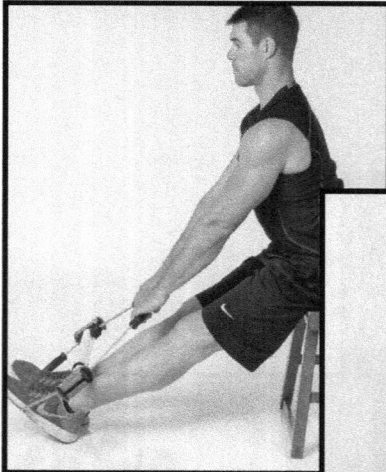

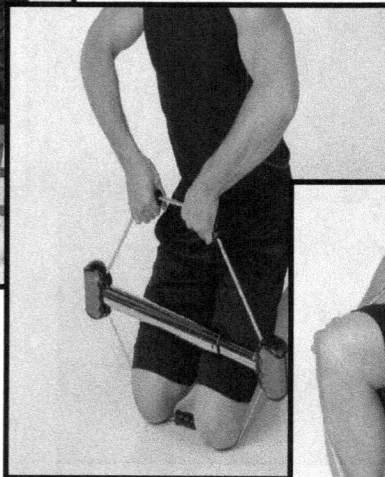

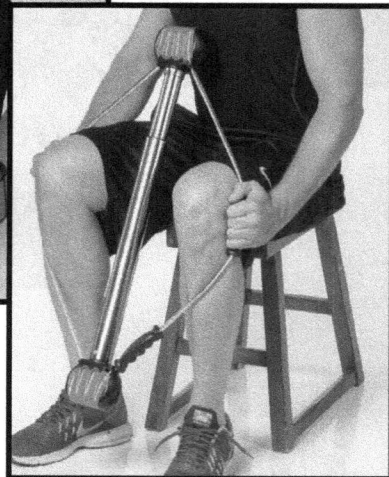

PHASE TWO

11 POWER REP RANGE X2 PHASE TWO

HOW TO PERFORM THIS ROUTINE:
POWER REP RANGE X2

Day 1=7-9 reps, Day 2=20 reps, Day 3=30 reps, Day 4=30 reps, Day 5=9 reps
Day 6=15 reps, Day 7=30 reps. On the last rep perform a 10 second
Isometric contraction. Perform all exercises without rest for 2 rounds.
Alternate day 1 and day 2......7 days per week for 4 weeks

DAY TWO continued...........

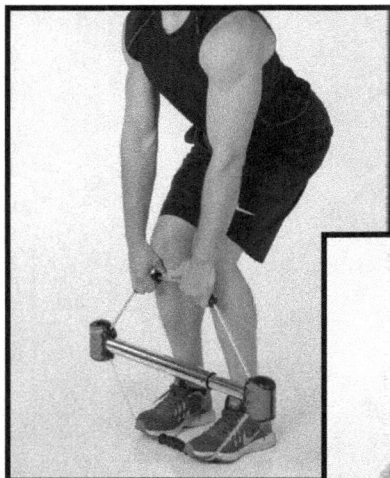

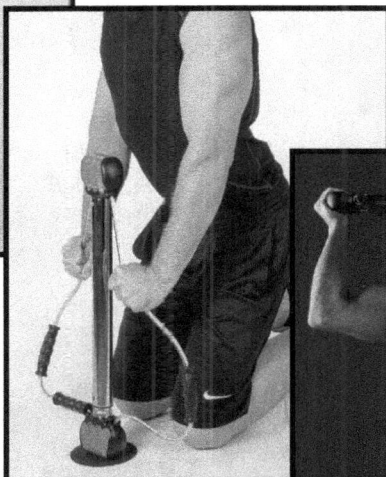

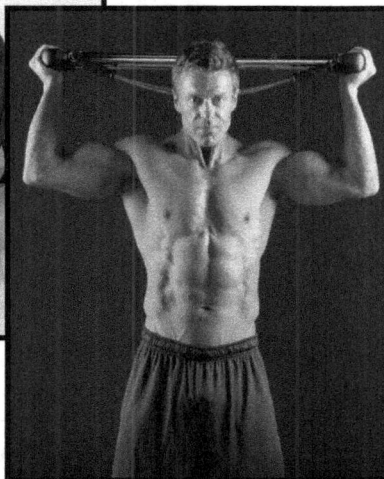

Looking forward to hearing from you on your progress. Please drop me an email skippymarl@icloud.com

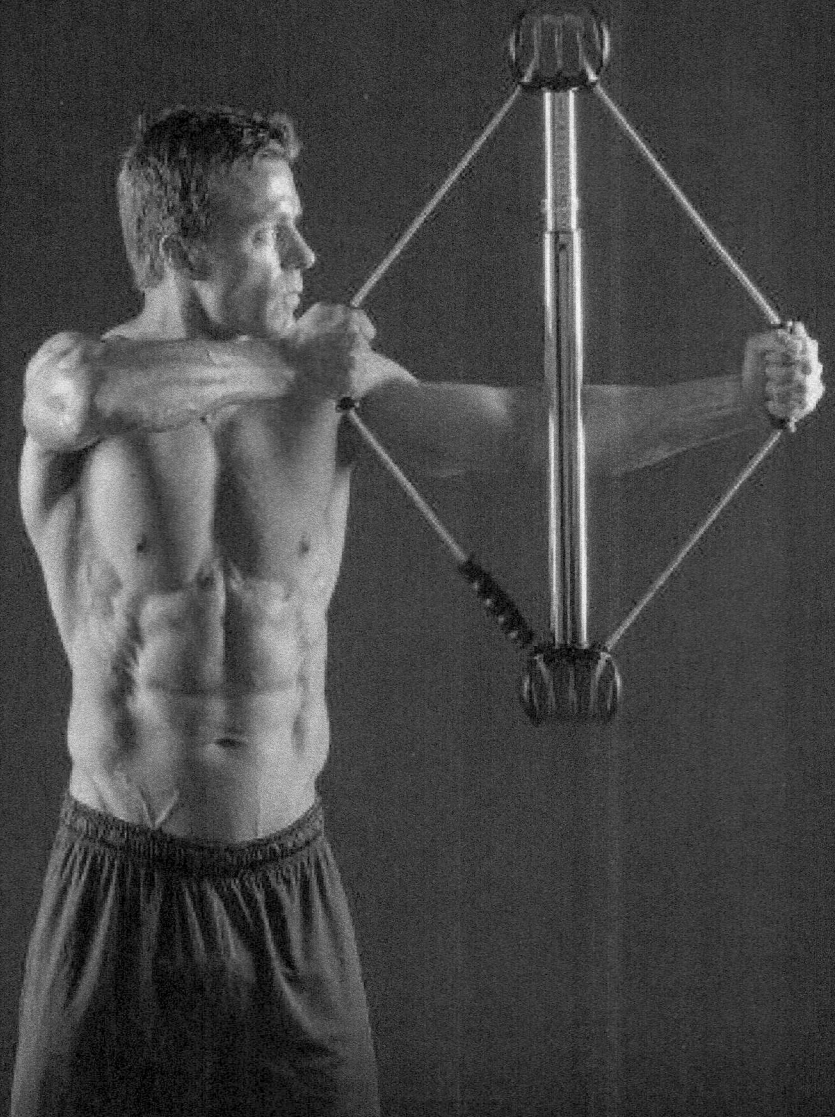

MOST IMPROVED STUDENT AWARD
COMING SOON
SEPTEMBER 31ST 2020

www.ingramcontent.com/pod-product-compliance
Lightning Source LLC
Chambersburg PA
CBHW081158270326
41930CB00014B/3207